Preface

The motivation for producing this book was derived from the enthusiasm of various teacher colleagues who have read an earlier publication *Functional Histology; a text and colour atlas*, Churchill Livingstone, Edinburgh (1979) of which two of us (P.R.W. and H.G.B.) were the principal authors. *Functional Histology* was aimed at medical and other university students specialising in biology; however, it has also found increasing use as a teaching manual by secondary school teachers. In this respect, *Functional Histology* is unnecessarily detailed and comprehensive for use by school students themselves and this book has, therefore, been prepared especially with their needs in mind.

This book is divided into three sections. The first section deals with the structure and function of the cell; in addition to the micrographs, mainly electron micrographs, the text and expanded captions cover all the major aspects of mammalian cytology required by A-level syllabuses. The second section introduces the basic tissue types, each chapter or new subsection commencing with a short introductory text summarising the main principles. The tissue types are then illustrated by appropriate colour micrographs, two and three dimensional diagrams and electron micrographs. The third section embraces the histology of the various organ systems, adopting a similar approach to that of the second section.

Wherever possible we have tried to avoid unnecessary jargon in the interests of simplicity. Throughout this work we have included ultrastructural details wherever it seemed to further understanding of the tissue structure and function. We make no apologies for covering some topics not yet established in school syllabuses, for example the immune system, in anticipation of their increasing importance in the future.

Nottingham

Paul Wheater
George Burkitt
Peter Lancaster

Acknowledgements

The authors are indebted to many individuals who have made invaluable contributions in their specialised fields.

Most of the tissue preparation and photomicrography was performed within the Departments of Pathology and Human Morphology of the Queen's Medical Centre, University of Nottingham. The authors are thus extremely grateful for the generous co-operation of Professors I. M. P. Dawson and R. E. Coupland. Special thanks are due to Mrs Janet Palmer of the Department of Pathology, who gave tireless assistance in the preparation of many of the tissues for light microscopy which were used in this book and many more preparations, for which space was not available. Similarly, our thanks are conveyed to Mr Paul Beck of the Department of Human Morphology for producing a large number of valuable specimens. Many of the electron micrographs were made available by Mr John Kugler and Mrs Annette Tomlinson, also of the Department of Human Morphology; to both we are deeply indebted.

Other people freely made available their resources: Mr Peter Crosby of the Department of Biology, University of York provided all the scanning electron micrographs, and his colleague Mr Brian Norman provided several light microscopic sections; Dr Robert Lang, also of York University, provided the freeze-etched preparation used in Figure 1.7; Mr Donald Canwell of the Physiological Laboratory, University of Cambridge contributed several sections from his personal collection; Dr Graham Robinson and Mr Stan Terras of the Department of Pathology, University of Nottingham each provided several electron micrographs, and they and their colleague, Miss Linda Burns, provided all the thin resin sections used for light microscopy; Dr David Tomlinson of the Department of Physiology, University of Nottingham contributed Figure 7.12; Dr Pat Cooke of the Department of Genetics, City Hospital, Nottingham lent the chromosome preparation used in Figure 2.2; Dr David Ansell of the Department of Pathology, City Hospital, Nottingham, Dr Hugh Rice and Dr Peter James of the Department of Pathology, Nottingham General Hospital, and Dr Pauline Cooper of the Department of Pathology, Addenbrooke's Hospital, Cambridge made available various tissue specimens and slides. Mr Peter Squires and Mr Hugh Pulsford of Huntingdon Research Centre, Cambridgeshire were a great source of help in providing the primate tissues used when suitable human tissues were unavailable. To all of these kind and co-operative people we express our sincere thanks.

Mr Bill Brackenbury of the Department of Pathology, University of Nottingham very skilfully performed all the macrophotography. All the remaining colour photomicrography was performed by one of the authors (P.R.W.). The onerous task of typing the manuscript was carried out with skill and great patience by Mrs Jane Richards.

P.R.W.
H.G.B.
P.L.

Colour Atlas of Histology 2.

,UTON SIXT

Paul R. Wheater
BA Hons (York), BMedSci Hons (Nott), BM BS (Nott)
The Queen's Medical Centre, University of Nottingham

H. George Burkitt
BD Sc Hons (Queensland), FRACDS, MMedSci (Nott),
MB BChir (Cantab)
School of Clinical Medicine, University of Cambridge

Peter Lancaster
BA Hons (York)
Biology Department, King Ecgbert School, Sheffield

Drawings by
Philip J. Deakin
BSc Hons (Sheff) MB ChB (Sheff)
The Medical School, University of Sheffield

LONGMAN

LONGMAN GROUP LIMITED
Longman House
Burnt Mill, Harlow, Essex CM20 2JE, England
and Associated Companies throughout the World

Distributed in the United States by Longman Inc,
1560 Broadway, New York, NY 10036

This edition first published by
Longman Group Limited 1985

ISBN 0 582 35269 X

Set in Monophoto Plantin 110

Produced by Longman Group (FE) Ltd.
Printed in Hong Kong.

Cover photomicrograph: Glands of the large intestine
(Alcian blue/Van Gieson stain)

Contents

Notes on staining techniques

1. Haematoxylin and eosin (H & E)

This is the most commonly used technique in animal histology and routine pathology. The basic dye haematoxylin stains acidic structures a purplish blue. Nuclei and rough endoplasmic reticulum, for example, both have a strong affinity for this dye owing to the high content of DNA and RNA respectively. In contrast, eosin is an acidic dye which stains basic structures red or pink. Most cytoplasmic proteins are basic and hence cytoplasm generally stains pink or pinkish red. In general, when the H & E staining technique is applied to animal cells, nuclei stain blue and cytoplasm stains pink or red.

2. Periodic acid–Schiff reaction (PAS)

Staining techniques which specifically stain components of cells and tissues are called histochemical staining techniques. Such techniques are invaluable for the understanding of cell and tissue structure and function, and for making a diagnosis on diseased tissues. The PAS reaction stains glycogen a deep red colour, traditionally described as magenta. The mucin produced by goblet cells of the gastro-intestinal and respiratory tracts stains magenta with this technique (and is therefore termed PAS positive). Basement membranes and the brush borders of kidney tubules and the small and large intestines are also PAS positive, as is cartilage and to some extent collagen.

3. Masson's trichrome

This technique is a so-called connective tissue technique since it is used to demonstrate connective tissue elements – principally collagen. As its name implies, the staining technique produces three colours; nuclei and other basophilic structures are stained blue, collagen is stained green or blue depending on which variant of the technique is used, and cytoplasm, muscle, erythrocytes and keratin are stained bright red.

4. Alcian blue

Alcian blue is a mucin stain which may be used in conjunction with other staining methods such as H & E or van Gieson (see below). Certain types of mucin, but not all, are stained blue by the Alcian blue method, as is cartilage. When the technique is combined with van Gieson, the Alcian blue colour becomes green.

5. Van Gieson

This is another connective tissue method in which collagen is stained red, nuclei blue and red cells and cytoplasm yellow. When used in combination with an elastic stain, elastin is stained blue/black in addition to the results described above. This staining technique is particularly useful for blood vessels and skin.

6. Reticulin stain

This method demonstrates the reticulin fibres of connective tissue which are stained blue/black by this technique. Nuclei may be counterstained blue with haematoxylin or red with the dye, neutral red.

7. Azan

This technique is traditionally classed as a connective tissue method but is excellent for demonstrating fine cytological detail, especially in epithelium. Nuclei are stained bright red; collagen, basement membrane and mucin are stained blue; muscle and red blood cells are stained orange to red.

8. Giemsa

This technique is a standard method for staining blood cells and other smears of cells. Nuclei are stained dark blue to violet, background cytoplasm pale blue and red cells pale pink.

9. Toluidine blue

This is a basic stain which stains acidic components various shades of blue. It is commonly employed on thin, resin-embedded specimens. Some tissue components are able to turn the blue dye red – a phenomenon known as metachromasia.

10. Silver and gold methods

These methods were extremely popular at the end of the nineteenth century and are occasionally used today to demonstrate such fine structures as cell processes (as in neurones), motor end-plates and intercellular junctions. Depending on the method used, the end product is either black, brown or golden.

11. Chrome alum haematoxylin

This method is rarely used and is similar to the H & E method in principle, in that nuclei are stained blue and cytoplasm is stained red. Empirically this method demonstrates the alpha cells of the pancreas as pink cells and the beta cells as blue.

12. Isamine blue/eosin

This method is also similar to the H & E method but the blue component is rather more intense.

13. Nissl and methylene blue methods

These techniques use a basic dye to stain the rough endoplasmic reticulum found in neurones: when this is seen as clumps it is called Nissl substance.

14. Sudan black and osmium

These dyes stain lipid-containing structures, such as myelin, a brownish-black colour.

Part A Cell structure, function and replication

Cell structure and function

Cell cycle and replication

1. Cell structure and function

Introduction

The cell, the functional unit of all tissues, has the capacity to perform individually all the essential life functions. Within the various tissues of the body, the constituent cells exhibit a wide range of specialisations which are, nevertheless, merely amplifications of one or more of the fundamental cellular processes. Reflecting their particular functional specialisations, mammalian cells have an extraordinary range of morphological forms yet all cells conform to a basic model of cell structure.

Even with primitive light microscopy, it was evident that cells were divided into at least two components, the *nucleus* and the *cytoplasm*, and as microscopical techniques advanced it became increasingly obvious that both the cytoplasm and the nucleus contained a number of subcellular elements which were called *organelles*. The advent of electron microscopy (EM) permitted description of the ultrastructure of these and many more organelles beyond the limit of resolution of the light microscope; the light microscope cannot resolve structures smaller than $0.5\,\mu m$ (500nm). Much of present knowledge about cell structure is based upon electron microscopy, but most cellular functions take place at the biochemical level which is even beyond the resolving capacity of the electron microscope; currently, structures smaller than about 1.0nm (10Å) are not generally resolvable. Microscopy is only one of many techniques which have been used to further the understanding of cell function and structure.

Fig. 1.1 The cell *(illustration opposite)*
(EM ×15000)

The basic organisational features common to all cells are illustrated in this electron micrograph of a hormone-secreting cell from the pituitary gland. All cells are bounded by an external limiting membrane called the *plasma membrane* or *plasmalemma* **PM** which serves as a dynamic interface between the internal environment of the cell and its various external environments. In this particular example, the cell interacts with two types of external environment: adjacent cells **C** and intercellular spaces **IS**.

The nucleus **N** is the largest organelle and its substance, often referred to as the *nucleoplasm*, is bounded by a membrane system called the *nuclear envelope* **NE**. The cytoplasm contains a variety of organelles most of which are also bounded by membranes. A diffuse system of membrane-bound tubules, saccules and flattened cisterns, collectively known as the *endoplasmic reticulum* **ER**, pervades the cytoplasm. A more distended system of membrane-bound saccules, the *Golgi apparatus* **G**, is usually found close to the nucleus. Scattered free in the cytoplasm are a number of relatively large, elongated organelles called *mitochondria* **M** which have a smooth outer membrane and a convoluted inner membrane system. In addition to these major organelles, the cell contains a variety of other membrane-bound structures, an example of which are the numerous, electron-dense *secretory vacuoles* **V** seen in this micrograph. Thus the cell is divided into a number of membrane-bound compartments each of which has its own particular biochemical environment. The organelles are suspended in a fluid medium called the *cytosol* which itself constitutes a discrete biochemical environment.

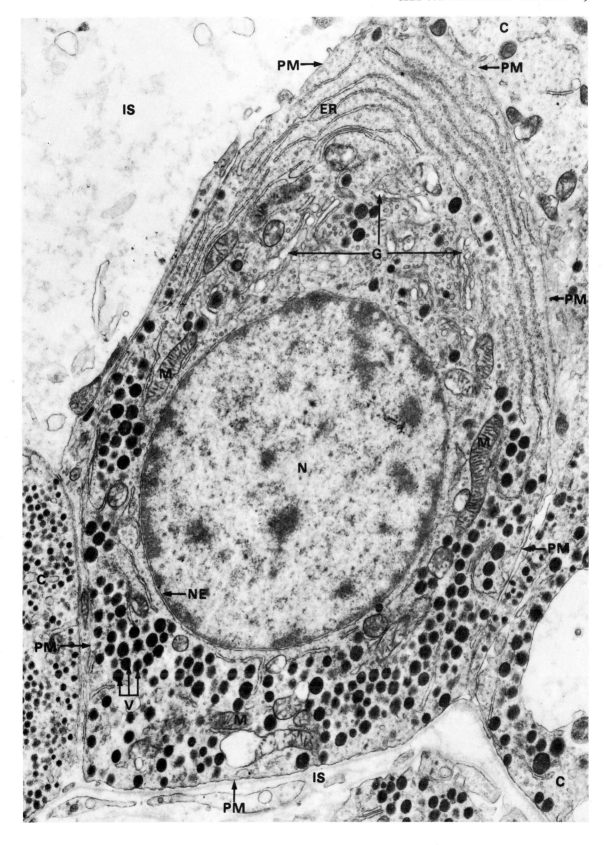

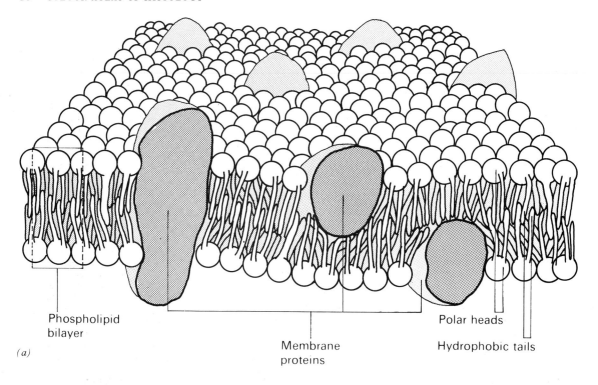

Phospholipid
bilayer

Membrane
proteins

Polar heads

Hydrophobic tails

(a)

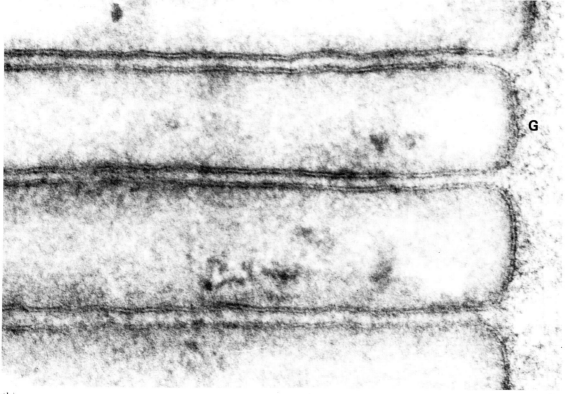

(b)

Fig. 1.2 Membrane structure

(a) Schematic diagram (b) EM × 330 000

Despite intensive investigation, the structure of cell membranes is still not known with certainty; however, a theoretical model has been progressively developed which satisfactorily incorporates much of the currently available biochemical and histological evidence.

Towards the end of the last century, it was observed that lipids rapidly gain entry into cells, and it was postulated that the 'cell boundary' was composed of lipid. In the 1920s it was found that, by measuring the minimum area that could be occupied by a monolayer of lipids extracted from a defined number of red blood cells, there was enough lipid present in the monolayer to cover each cell twice. From this it was concluded that the cells were bounded by a double layer of lipid. Later, it was proposed that cell membranes are symmetrical structures consisting of a bilayer of phospholipid molecules sandwiched between two layers of protein. This model, however, failed to explain the selective permeability of most cell membranes to molecules which are not lipid soluble such as glucose, sodium ions and potassium ions. These difficulties were theoretically overcome by postulating the existence of 'pores' composed of protein, through which hydrophilic molecules could readily be transported by passive or active mechanisms. As a result of electron microscopic studies in the late 1950s, the concept of the 'unit membrane' was devised, in which it was envisaged that all cell membranes have the same structure, since they all appeared to have the same trilaminate ultrastructure.

The current concepts of membrane structure are shown diagrammatically (opposite). In this model, cell membranes are considered to consist of a bilayer of phospholipid molecules; the hydrophilic (lipid-insoluble) portions of the phospholipid molecules of each layer are aggregated at the surface with their hydrophobic 'tails' projecting into the centre of the membrane where they interact with the hydrophobic 'tails' of the opposed phospholipid layer. The weak intermolecular forces which hold the bilayer together allow individual molecules of phospholipid to move relatively freely within each layer. Cell membranes are therefore highly fluid in nature, yet have the ordered structure of a crystal. Cholesterol molecules are incorporated in the hydrophobic regions of the membrane and modify the fluidity of the membrane. In this model, proteins are scattered in the phospholipid bilayer, some of them extending through the entire thickness of the membrane to be exposed to each surface; it is proposed that these molecules function as 'pores' through which hydrophilic molecules are transported either passively or actively. These proteins, and others which do not span the whole width of the membrane, are also freely mobile within the plane of the phospholipid bilayer. This model is known as the *'fluid mosaic model'* of membrane structure.

On the external surface of the plasma membranes of animal cells, many of the membrane proteins and some of the membrane lipids are conjugated with short chains of polysaccharide; these glycoproteins and glycolipids project from the surface of the bilayer forming an outer coating which may be analogous to the cell walls of plants, bacteria and fungi. This polysaccharide layer has been termed the *glycocalyx* and appears to vary in thickness in different cell types; whether an analogous layer exists on all membranes or only at the external surface is unknown. The function of the glycocalyx is obscure, but there is evidence that it may be involved in cell recognition phenomena, in the formation of intercellular adhesions, and in the adsorption of molecules to the cell surface. Alternatively, the glycocalyx may simply provide mechanical and chemical protection for the plasma membrane.

The electron micrograph in (b) provides a high magnification view of a plasma membrane; this example illustrates the minute surface projections of a lining cell from the small intestine. All membranes have a characteristic trilaminate appearance comprising two electron-dense layers separated by an electron-lucent layer. The outer dense layers are thought to correspond to the hydrophilic 'heads' of phospholipid molecules whilst the electron-lucent layer is thought to represent the intermediate hydrophobic layer mainly consisting of fatty acid side chains. On the external surface of the plasma membrane an outer fibrillar coat, called the *'fuzzy coat'*, represents the glycocalyx **G**. This is an unusually prominent feature of small intestinal lining cells.

Transport across plasma membranes

Plasma membranes mediate the continuous exchange of metabolites between the internal and external environments of the cell in four principal ways. These mechanisms enable the cell to control the quality of its internal environment with a high degree of specificity.

(i) Passive diffusion: this type of transport is entirely dependent on the presence of a concentration gradient across the plasma membrane. Lipids and lipid-soluble metabolites such as ethanol pass freely through plasma membranes; plasma membranes also offer little barrier to the diffusion of gases such as oxygen and carbon dioxide. The plasma membrane is, in general, impermeable to hydrophilic molecules; nevertheless some small molecules including water and urea, and inorganic ions such as bicarbonate, are able to pass down osmotic or electrochemical gradients through the membrane via hydrophilic regions, the nature of which remains obscure.

(ii) Facilitated diffusion: this type of transport is also concentration-dependent and involves the transport of larger hydrophilic metabolites such as glucose and amino-acids. The process is strictly passive but requires the presence of so-called 'carriers' to which the metabolites bind specifically but reversibly in a manner analogous to the binding of substrate with enzyme.

(iii) Active transport: this mode of transport is not only independent of concentration gradients but also often operates against extreme concentration gradients. The classical example of this form of transport is the continuous transport of sodium out of the cell by the so-called 'sodium pump'; this process requires the expenditure of energy provided in the form of ATP. It is postulated that this form of transport occurs through 'dynamic pores' consisting of proteins or protein systems which span the plasma membrane. Both active and passive transport processes are enhanced by increasing the area of the plasma membrane by folds or projections of the cell surface as exemplified by the absorptive cells lining the small intestine (see Fig. 1.2).

(iv) Bulk transport: bulk transport involves engulfment of large molecules or small particles by cytoplasmic extensions, thus forming membrane-bound vacuoles within the cytoplasm. When this process involves the creation of small vacuoles it is known as *pinocytosis*, and when large vacuoles are formed it is called *phagocytosis*. The term *endocytosis*, encompassing both processes, is probably a more appropriate term for bulk transport into the cell. Endocytotic vesicles either discharge their contents directly into the cytoplasm or fuse with membrane-bound organelles called *lysosomes*; lysosomes contain more than twelve different enzymes which are capable of degrading carbohydrates, lipids, proteins, nucleic acids and other organic molecules. Lysosomal enzymes digest engulfed material which is then made available for metabolic processes. In many secretory processes, bulk transport also occurs in the opposite direction when it is termed *exocytosis*.

Histologically, the passive and active processes of transport can only be observed indirectly; for example, cells suspended in hypotonic solutions swell due to passive uptake of water whereas cells placed in hypertonic solutions tend to shrink due to outflow of water. Radio-isotope labelling techniques can be used to follow active transport processes. Bulk transport, however, is readily observable by microscopy.

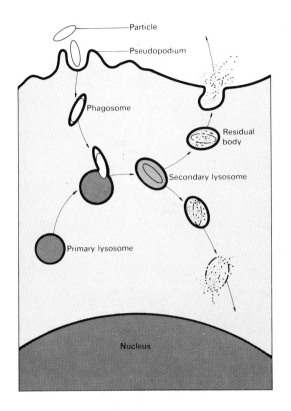

Fig. 1.3 Endocytosis

This diagram summarises the main steps in endocytosis of particulate matter. The first stage of phagocytosis involves recognition of a particle; this then becomes surrounded by cytoplasmic extensions called *pseudopodia*. When the particle is completely surrounded, the plasma membrane fuses and the membrane surrounding the engulfed particle forms a vesicle, known as a *phagosome* or *endocytotic vesicle*, which detaches from the plasma membrane to float freely within the cytoplasm. The phagosome is then in some way recognised by one or more *primary lysosomes* which fuse with the phagosome to form a *secondary lysosome*. This exposes the engulfed material to a battery of lysosomal enzymes. When digestion is complete, the lysosomal membrane may rupture, discharging its contents into the cytoplasm. Undigested material may remain within membrane-bound vesicles called *residual bodies*, the contents of which may be discharged at the cell surface by exocytosis; alternatively residual bodies may accumulate in the cytoplasm.

Lysosomes are also involved in the degradation of cellular organelles, many of which have only a finite lifespan and are therefore replaced continuously; this lysosomal function is termed *autophagy*. Most autophagocytic degradation products are reutilised by the cell, but some indigestible products accumulate and become indistinguishable from the residual bodies of endocytosis. With advancing age, residual bodies accumulate in the cells of some tissues and appear as brown so-called *lipofuscin granules*.

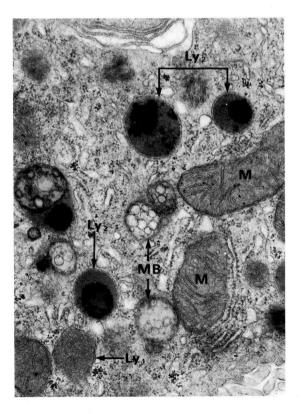

Fig. 1.4 Lysosomes

(EM × 27000)

This micrograph shows the typical appearance of lysosomes in the cytoplasm of a liver cell. Primary lysosomes Ly_1 vary greatly in size and appearance but they are recognised as membrane-bound organelles containing a granular, amorphous material. Secondary lysosomes Ly_2 are even more variable in appearance but are recognisable by their diverse particulate content some of which is extremely electron-dense. The distinction between residual bodies and secondary lysosomes is often difficult, but one distinctive type of residual body, the so-called *multivesicular body* **MB**, is seen in this micrograph. Multivesicular bodies are membrane-bound vesicles containing a number of smaller vesicles which are thought to represent the debris of cell membrane degradation. Note the size of lysosomes relative to mitochondria **M**.

Protein synthesis

Proteins are not only a major structural component of cells but, in the form of enzymes, mediate every metabolic process within the cell. Thus the nature and quantity of proteins present within any individual cell determines the activity of that cell. Both the structural proteins and enzymes of the cell are subject to wear and tear and are replaced continuously. Many cells also synthesise proteins for export; such proteins include glandular secretions and extracellular structural components of tissues. Protein synthesis is, therefore, an essential and continuous activity of all cells and the major function of some cells.

The principal organelles involved in protein synthesis are the *nucleus* and *ribosomes*. The nucleus of every cell contains within its complement of DNA a template for each protein that can be made by that individual as a whole. However, most cells only synthesise a certain defined range of proteins which are characteristic of the particular cell type and therefore only part of the DNA template is utilised. The process of protein synthesis involves *transcription* of the DNA code for a particular protein by synthesis of the specific, complementary messenger RNA (mRNA) molecule. The mRNA molecule then enters the cytoplasm to associate with ribosomes upon which protein synthesis occurs; the amino-acid sequence of the resulting protein is determined by *translation* of the mRNA code.

Ribosomes are minute cytoplasmic organelles, each composed of two subunits of unequal size. Each subunit consists of a strand of RNA (ribosomal RNA) with associated ribosomal proteins; the ribosomal RNA strand and associated proteins are folded to form a condensed, globular structure. Ribosomes are highly active structures with specific receptor proteins which align mRNA strands so that transfer RNA (tRNA) molecules carrying the appropriate amino-acids may be brought into position prior to the addition of their amino-acids to the growing polypeptide chain. Other ribosomal proteins are involved in catalysing peptide bond formation between amino-acids. Individual ribosomes are too small to be clearly resolved by electron microscopy although they are visible as small electron-dense masses at high magnification; nevertheless, the detail of ribosome structure and function are well established at the molecular level. Ribosomes are found free in the cytoplasm either singly or as small aggregations called *polyribosomes* or *polysomes*; ribosomes are also attached to the surface of the extensive intra-cytoplasmic membrane system known as the endoplasmic reticulum (see Fig. 1.8).

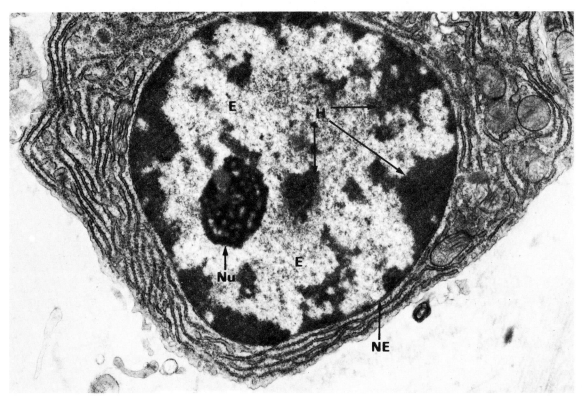

Fig. 1.5 Nucleus

(EM × 15 400)

This micrograph illustrates the typical nucleus of a highly active, protein-secreting cell. The nuclear envelope **NE**, separating the nuclear contents from the cytoplasm, is barely visible at this magnification. The nucleus not only contains DNA, which comprises less than twenty per cent of its mass, but also contains a large quantity of protein called *nucleoprotein*, and some RNA. Most of the nucleoprotein is intimately associated with DNA; the remainder consists of enzymes responsible for RNA and DNA synthesis. The nuclear RNA represents newly synthesised messenger, transfer and ribosomal RNA which has not yet passed into the cytoplasm.

Except during cell division, the chromosomes, each comprising a discrete length of the DNA complement, exist as tangled strands which extend throughout the nucleus and cannot be visualised individually by direct electron microscopy. Nuclei appear as heterogeneous structures with electron-dense and electron-lucent areas. The dense areas, called *heterochromatin*, represent that portion of the DNA complement and its associated nucleoprotein which is not active in protein synthesis. Heterochromatin **H** tends.to be clumped around the periphery of the nucleus but also forms irregular clumps throughout the nucleus. In females, the quiescent X-chromosome (equivalent to the Y-chromosome of the male) forms a small discrete mass known as a *Barr body*; Barr bodies are seen at the edge of the nucleus in a small proportion of female cells when cut in a favourable plane of section. The electron-lucent nuclear material, called *euchromatin* **E**, represents that part of the DNA which is active in protein synthesis. Collectively, heterochromatin and euchromatin are known as *chromatin*, a name derived from the strongly coloured appearance of nuclei when stained for light microscopy.

Many nuclei, especially those of cells highly active in protein synthesis, contain one or more extremely dense structures called *nucleoli* **Nu** which are the sites of ribosomal RNA synthesis. Each cell type has a characteristic nucleolar morphology. In general, the degree of activity of any cell may be judged by the ultrastructural appearance of its nucleus. Relatively inactive cells have small nuclei in which the chromatin is predominantly in the condensed form (heterochromatin) and in which the nucleolus is small or absent.

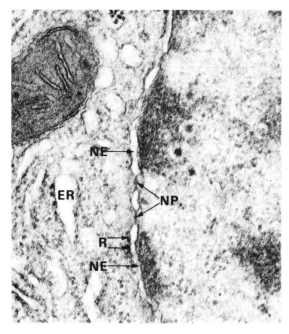

Fig. 1.6 Nuclear envelope
(EM × 67 500)

The nuclear envelope **NE** consists of two layers of membrane. The space between these layers is known to be continuous, in places, with cisternae of the endoplasmic reticulum; thus the nuclear envelope may be considered as a specialised region of the endoplasmic reticulum. Like the endoplasmic reticulum **ER**, the outer surface of the outer nuclear membrane is often studded with ribosomes **R**. A considerable proportion of the nuclear envelope contains apparent perforations called *nuclear pores* **NP**, at the margins of which the inner and outer membranes become continuous. The membrane at the periphery of each pore is thickened and each pore appears to be closed by a diaphragm of unknown structure. Nuclear pores may permit the exchange of metabolites between the nucleus and cytoplasm; it is suggested that the pores are the sites through which RNA molecules enter the cytoplasm.

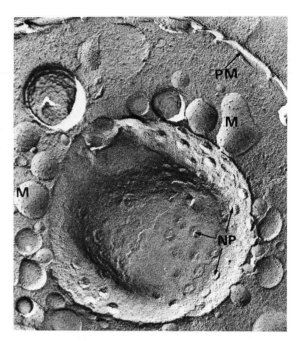

Fig. 1.7 Nuclear pores
(Freeze-etched preparation × 34000)

This micrograph shows an example of a technique called *freeze-etching*. Briefly, this method involves the rapid cooling of cells to subzero temperatures; the frozen cells are then fractured. This exposes internal surfaces of the cell in a somewhat random manner although the fracture lines tend to follow natural planes of weakness. Further surface detail is obtained by 'etching' or subliming excess water molecules from the specimen at low temperature. A thin carbon impression is then made of the surface and this mirror image is viewed by conventional electron microscopy. Freeze-etching provides a valuable tool for studying internal cell surfaces at high resolution.

In this preparation, the plane of cleavage has included part of the nuclear envelope and nuclear pores **NP** are clearly demonstrated. Note also the outline of the plasma membrane **PM** and mitochondria **M**.

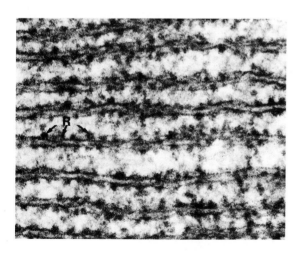

Fig. 1.8 Rough endoplasmic reticulum
(EM × 103 400)

As previously described, the endoplasmic reticulum consists of an anastomosing network of tubules, vesicles and flattened cisternae which ramifies throughout the cytoplasm. Much of the surface of the endoplasmic reticulum is studded with ribosomes **R** giving the reticulum a rough or granular appearance; such endoplasmic reticulum is therefore called *rough* or *granular endoplasmic reticulum* (rER or gER). This micrograph illustrates rough ER in a cell which is specialised for the synthesis and secretion of protein; in such cells, rough ER tends to be profuse and to form closely packed, parallel laminae of flattened cisternae. It has been proposed that protein is synthesised on the ribosomes of the external surface of rough ER and then passed into the cisternal cavity; the interconnected cisternal cavities may act as intracellular pathways for the transport of newly synthesised protein.

Lipid biosynthesis

Lipids are synthesised by all cells in order to repair and replace damaged or worn membranes. Many cells also synthesise lipid as a means of storing excess energy; in such cells lipid is stored as cytoplasmic droplets. The synthesis of all classes of lipid is based on the precursor molecules fatty acids, triglycerides and cholesterol. These precursors are available to the cell from dietary sources or as a result of mobilisation of lipid stores in other cells. Fatty acids, triglycerides and cholesterol, however, can be synthesised by most cells using simple sources of carbon such as acetyl-CoA and other intermediates of glucose catabolism. Fatty acids and triglycerides are mostly synthesised within the cytosol, whereas cholesterol and phospholipids are synthesised in areas of endoplasmic reticulum devoid of ribosomes called *smooth endoplasmic reticulum* (sER). Cells which are highly active in lipid biosynthesis, such as liver cells, tend to have well developed networks of smooth ER.

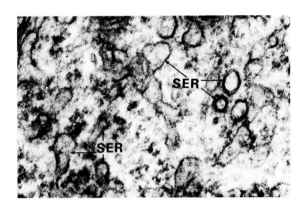

Fig. 1.9 Smooth endoplasmic reticulum
(EM × 92 400)

This micrograph shows part of the prolific smooth ER **SER** of a steroid hormone secreting cell; steroid hormones are lipids derived from the precursor cholesterol. Smooth ER usually consists of an irregular network of tubules and vesicles rather than flattened cisternae as in rough ER. In addition to its role in lipid biosynthesis, smooth ER is also thought to be part of the intracellular transport system since it is continuous with rough ER and with the Golgi apparatus (see Fig. 1.11). A modified form of smooth ER is present in nerve and muscle cells (see Chapters 5 and 7) where it is believed to have specialised storage and transport functions.

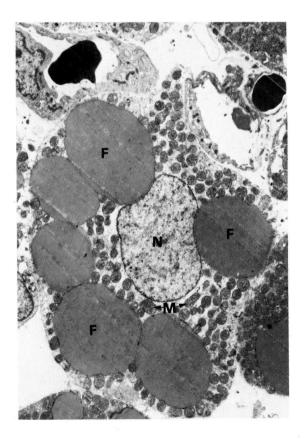

Fig. 1.10 Lipid storage
(EM × 4070)

This micrograph illustrates multiple cytoplasmic fat droplets **F**; note their size relative to the cell nucleus **N** and that they are not membrane bound. This example is from brown adipose tissue, a highly specialised form of fat tissue found mainly in newborn and hibernating mammals; such animals must be capable of releasing energy rapidly, immediately after birth and at the end of hibernation respectively. Note the numerous mitochondria **M** which are involved in energy release by uncoupling of oxidative phosphorylation from the electron transfer chain.

Secretion

The export from cells of materials, which may be excretory waste products or secretory products, involves the four principal mechanisms outlined earlier for the transport of materials into cells. Excretion or secretion of small molecular weight compounds or lipid-soluble materials rarely involves bulk transport, whereas secretion of proteins and protein complexes almost exclusively involves bulk transport. Prior to release from the cell, proteins and other secretory products are packaged within membrane-bound vesicles which then fuse with the surface plasma membrane thus releasing their contents by the process of exocytosis. The Golgi apparatus (also called *Golgi body* or *Golgi complex*) is the organelle primarily responsible for the packaging process. During the secretory process in highly secretory cells, large amounts of intracellular membrane become incorporated into the plasma membrane; there must be, therefore, a complementary mechanism for reabsorbing excess plasma membrane and returning it to the internal pool of membrane.

An unexplained finding is that certain cell types have a well developed Golgi apparatus but are manifestly not involved in secretory activities. A possible explanation for this finding may be that the primary function of the Golgi apparatus in all cells is the production of new membrane necessary for cell growth and to replace membrane lost or damaged during normal metabolic activities; the well established packaging role of the Golgi apparatus may represent a specialisation of the suggested primary function.

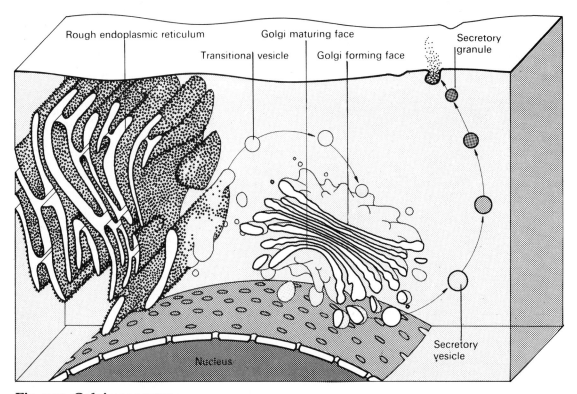

Fig. 1.11 Golgi apparatus

This schematic diagram illustrates the main structural features of the Golgi apparatus and summarises the probable mechanism by which secretory products are packaged within membrane-bound vesicles. The Golgi apparatus consists of a stacked system of saucer-shaped cisternae, with the concave surface facing the nucleus. Proteins, synthesised on ribosomes of the rough ER, are transported within the endoplasmic reticulum to the region of the Golgi apparatus. Membrane-bound vesicles containing protein, known as *transitional vesicles*, bud off from the endoplasmic reticulum and then coalesce with the convex surface of the Golgi apparatus, an area of the Golgi

apparatus known as the *forming face*. By a mechanism still unresolved, secretory product is passed towards the concave surface, the *maturing face*, where new vesicles containing secretory product are formed. Some proteinaceous secretion products consist of protein-carbohydrate complexes; it is known that the carbohydrate component is added during passage through the Golgi apparatus. After release from the maturing face the contents of *secretory vesicles* become condensed to form mature secretory vesicles, often termed *secretory granules*, which are then liberated at the cell surface by exocytosis.

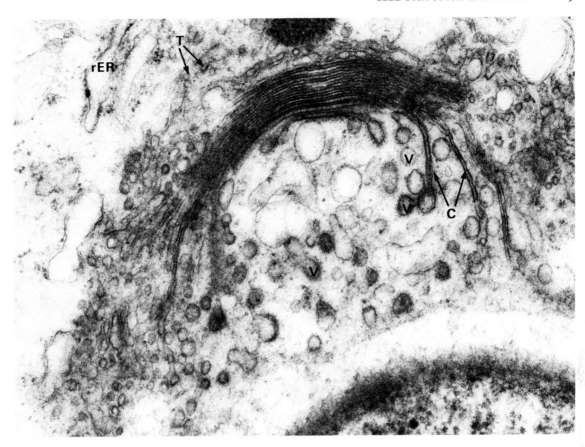

Fig. 1.12 Golgi apparatus

(EM ×49950)

The Golgi apparatus is a dynamically changing structure, the appearance of which varies enormously according to the functional state of the cell; for this reason the 'classical' appearance of the Golgi apparatus is, in practice, rarely seen. This micrograph illustrates a particularly well developed Golgi apparatus; transitional vesicles **T** and elements of the rough endoplasmic reticulum **rER** are seen adjacent to the forming face. A variety of larger vesicles **V** can be seen in the concavity of the maturing face, some of which appear to be budding from the Golgi cisternae **C**. A large number of intermediate vesicles can be seen close to the periphery of the cisternal stack. Note the proximity of the Golgi apparatus to the nucleus **N** and its orientation with the forming face directed towards the nucleus.

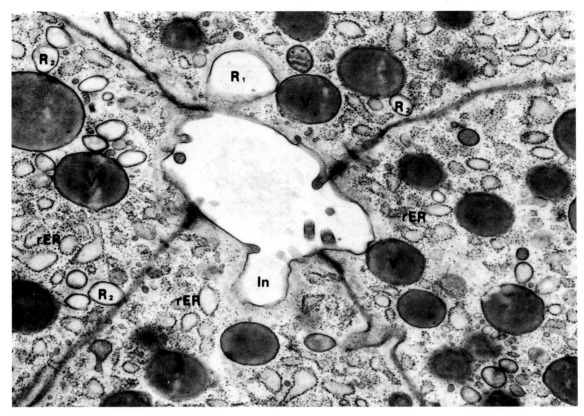

Fig. 1.13 Exocytosis

(EM ×28900)

This micrograph shows the apical regions of four secretory cells converging on a central channel. Large, membrane-bound secretory vesicles **V** are seen approaching the lumen, one of which appears to be fusing with the surface plasma membrane. A deep invagination **In** in one of the plasma membranes probably represents a secretory vesicle which has just discharged its contents. Although the fate of membrane from discharged vesicles is not clear, a large vesicle R_1, and numerous smaller, apparently empty vesicles R_2 may represent vesicle membrane in the process of being recycled. Note also in this micrograph a well developed system of rough endoplasmic reticulum **rER** with dilated cisternae; numerous free ribosomes are present in the cytoplasm.

Energy production and storage

All cellular functions are dependent on a continuous supply of energy. Energy is derived from the sequential breakdown of organic molecules during the process of *cellular respiration*; the energy released from the breakage of chemical bonds during this process is ultimately stored in the form of ATP molecules. In actively respiring cells, ATP forms a pool of readily available energy for all the metabolic functions of the cell. The main substrates for cellular respiration are simple sugars and lipids, particularly glucose and fatty acids. Cellular respiration of glucose begins in the cytosol where it is partially degraded to form pyruvic acid by the process known as glycolysis, which yields a small amount of ATP. Pyruvic acid then diffuses into specialised organelles called *mitochondria* where, in the presence of oxygen, it is degraded to carbon dioxide and water in a process which yields a large quantity of ATP. In contrast, fatty acids pass directly into mitochondria where they are also degraded to carbon dioxide and water; this process also yields a large amount of ATP. Glycolysis may occur in the absence of oxygen and is therefore termed anaerobic respiration, whereas mitochondrial respiration is dependent on a continuous supply of oxygen and is therefore termed aerobic respiration. Mitochondria are the principal organelles involved in cellular respiration in mammals, and are found in large numbers in metabolically active cells as in the liver.

Under favourable nutritional conditions, most cells generate and store excess glucose and fatty acids in the relatively insoluble and non-toxic forms glycogen and triglyceride respectively. Cells vary greatly in their content of stored carbohydrate and lipid; extreme examples are nerve cells which contain almost no intracellular glycogen or triglyceride, and fat cells, the cytoplasm of which is almost entirely filled with stored lipid.

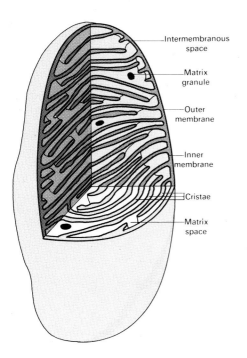

Intermembranous space

Matrix granule

Outer membrane

Inner membrane

Cristae

Matrix space

Fig. 1.14 Mitochondrion

Mitochondria vary enormously in size and shape but are most often elongated, cigar-shaped organelles. Each mitochondrion consists of two layers of membrane; the inner membrane is thrown into folds, called *cristae*, projecting into the inner cavity which is filled with an amorphous substance called *matrix*. The matrix contains a number of dense *matrix granules* the nature and function of which are unclear. The inner mitochondrial membrane is closely applied to the outer membrane leaving a narrow intermembranous space which extends into each crista.

Aerobic respiration takes place within the matrix and inner mitochondrial membranes. The matrix contains most of the enzymes involved in oxidation of fatty acids and the enzymes of the tricarboxylic acid cycle (Krebs cycle). The inner membrane contains the cytochromes, the carrier molecules of the electron transport chain, and the enzymes involved in ATP production. There is evidence that these molecules are arranged in an ordered manner as discrete functional units called *respiratory assemblies* within the mitochondrial inner membrane, but whether these units have a structure which is discernible with the electron microscope is in dispute.

Mitochondria, as organelles, have several most unusual features. The mitochondrial matrix contains a strand of DNA arranged as a circle in a manner analogous to the chromosomes of bacteria. The matrix also contains ribosomes which have a similar structure to bacterial ribosomes. There is evidence that mitochondria synthesise at least some of their own constituent proteins, others being synthesised by the cell in which they reside. In addition, mitochondria undergo self-replication by a process which is similar to bacterial cell division. On the basis of these features, it has been proposed that mitochondria are semi-autonomous organelles which arose during evolution as bacterial intracellular parasites of larger, more advanced cells.

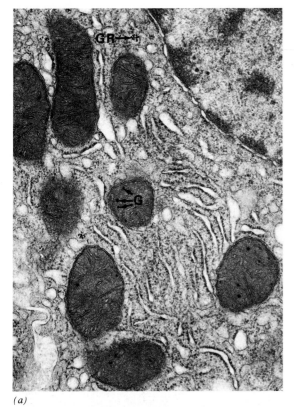

(a)

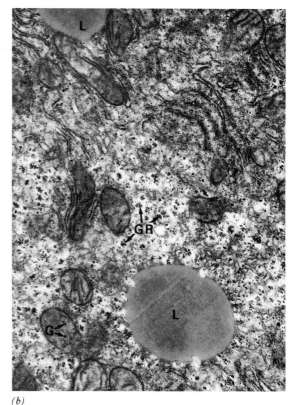

(b)

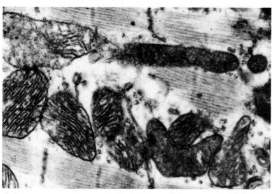

(c)

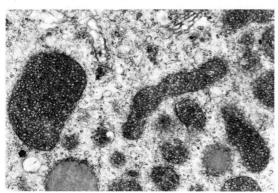

(d)

Fig. 1.15 Mitochondria, lipid droplets and glycogen

(EM (a) ×21 200 (b) ×18 200 (c) ×21 300 (d) ×16 200)

All mitochondria conform to the same general structure but vary greatly in size, shape and arrangement of cristae; these variations often reflect the metabolic status of the cell type in which mitochondria are found. Mitochondria move freely within the cytosol and tend to aggregate in intracellular sites with high energy demands where their shape often conforms to the available space. Micrographs (a) and (b), both of liver cell cytoplasm, show the typical appearance of mitochondria when cut in different planes of section; note the relatively dense matrix containing a few matrix granules **G**. Glycogen and lipid droplets are also seen in (a) and (b); glycogen appears either as single, minute dense granules (called α *particles*) or as aggregations termed *glycogen rosettes* **GR**, also called β *particles*. Lipid droplets **L** are of variable size and electron density and are not bounded by a membrane. Mitochondria from heart muscle and steroid-secreting cells can be seen in (c) and (d) respectively; in each, the cristae are densely packed, reflecting the metabolic activity of the cell, and have a characteristic shape. The cristae of heart muscle mitochondria are laminar whereas those of steroid-secreting cells are tubular.

The cytoskeleton and cell movement

The concept of a *cytoskeleton* has been evolved to explain how cell shape is maintained and altered during such processes as endocytosis, amoeboid movement and cell division. The cytoskeleton is thought to consist of an internal framework of minute filaments and tubules which may not only provide structural support but also may direct intracellular movement of organelles and metabolites. Cell movement would thus depend on rearrangement of the supporting elements, a process termed *contractility*. In muscle cells, which are highly specialised contractile cells, the contractile mechanism is thought to involve the movement of minute filaments relative to one another, according to the *sliding filament theory* (see Fig. 6.7), but this mechanism may not be wholly applicable to all cell types.

The minute filaments of the cytoskeleton, called *microfilaments*, are probably a mixed population of filamentous proteins of which the protein *actin* is the major constituent. Since actin is known to be one of the major filament types involved in muscle contraction, it may have a similar role in the cytoskeleton of other cell types. In some cells, microfilaments are arranged as bundles called *tonofibrils*; tonofibrils appear to converge upon the plasma membrane in the region of certain types of intercellular junctions (see Fig. 1.19) thus integrating the plasma membrane into the cytoskeleton.

The tubular structures of the cytoskeleton, *microtubules*, are demonstrable in the cytoplasm of many cell types where they may provide the major elements of a supporting framework. Microtubules are composed of subunits of a globular protein called *tubulin* arranged in a closely packed, helical manner. Tubulin subunits appear to disaggregate and reaggregate readily, thereby providing a dynamic, rather than static, framework.

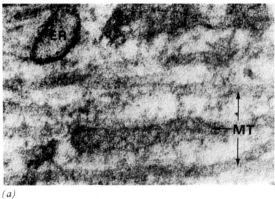

(a)   *(b)*

Fig. 1.16 Microtubules

(EM (a) LS × 171 500 (b) TS × 171 500)

These micrographs illustrate microtubules within nerve cells; each nerve cell has an extremely elongated cytoplasmic extension called an axon (see Chapter 7) in which microtubules are unusually prominent. The axonal microtubules probably provide structural support and direct intra-axonal transport. In longitudinal section, microtubules **MT** appear as straight, unbranched structures and in transverse section appear hollow. The small diameter

of microtubules is evident when compared with an adjacent small mitochondrion **M** and elements of smooth endoplasmic reticulum **ER**. Microtubules may direct intracellular transport by acting as 'guide rails' for the movement of organelles such as mitochondria or secretory vesicles; alternatively microtubules may merely act as a system of internal tubes for conveying molecules within the cytoplasm.

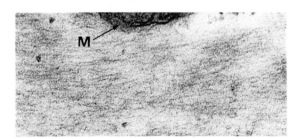

Fig. 1.17 Microfilaments

(EM × 76 500)

In general, individual microfilaments are difficult to demonstrate because of their small diameter and diffuse arrangement amongst other cytoplasmic components. In this example from a smooth muscle cell, a cell type in which cytoplasmic filaments are a predominant feature, parallel arrays of microfilaments are readily seen. The diameter of microfilaments may be compared with the size of a mitochondrion **M**.

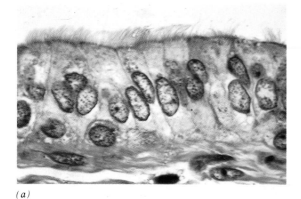

(a)

Fig. 1.18 Cilia

(a) Bronchiolar epithelium (resin embedded, one micron section: toluidine blue × 800)
(b) Schematic diagram of a cilium
(c) Scanning EM × 2000

Cilia are motile structures which project in parallel rows from some epithelial surface cells. Cilia measure from about 7–10 μm in length and may therefore be of the order of half the length of the cell depending on cell size. A single epithelial cell may have up to 300 cilia and these are usually about the same length. Cilia beat with a wavelike, synchronous rhythm which tends to propel surface films of mucus or fluid in a consistent direction over the epithelial surface.

Each cilium, which is bounded by an evagination of the luminal plasma membrane, contains a central core called the *axoneme* consisting of twenty microtubules arranged as a central pair surrounded by nine peripheral doublets. Near the cytoplasmic surface, each axoneme inserts into a structure called a *basal body* which has a microtubular arrangement identical to that of a centriole; that is, nine triplets of microtubules forming a short cylinder (see Fig. 2.6). Each peripheral doublet of the cilium axoneme continues into the two inner microtubules of the corresponding triplet of the basal body. The central pair of axoneme microtubules terminates outside the basal body. Note that each axoneme doublet consists of one tubule, which is circular in cross section, closely applied to another incomplete tubule which is C-shaped in cross-section. From each complete tubule, pairs of 'arms' consisting of the protein *dynein*, which has ATP-ase activity, extend towards the incomplete tubule of the adjacent doublet. It is believed that ciliary action results from longitudinal movement of the doublets relative to one another, energy for the process being provided in the form of ATP probably by mitochondria which crowd the subjacent cytoplasm. It is not yet clear whether basal bodies arise *de novo* or by repeated division of centrioles. Note that evidence of basal bodies can be seen even with light microscopy. A three-dimensional surface view of cilia in the respiratory tract is shown in micrograph (c).

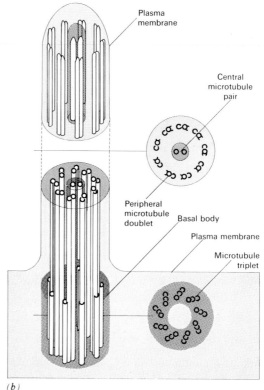

(b)

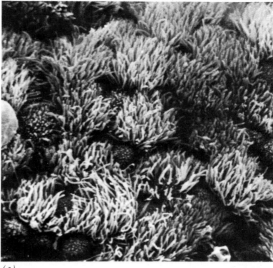

(c)

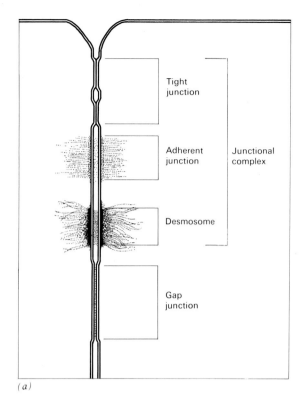

(a)

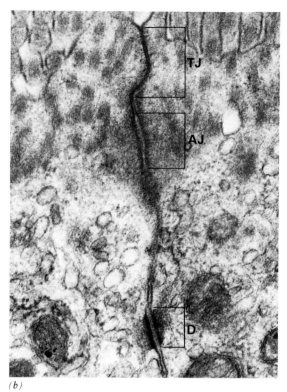

(b)

Fig. 1.19 Cell junctions

(a) Schematic diagram
(b) Junctional complex (EM × 59 400)

Before the advent of electron microscopy, epithelial cells were thought to be bound together by an intercellular adhesive which was called *intercellular cement*. It is now known that epithelial cells are bound together by several types of plasma membrane specialisations to which a variety of somewhat confusing names have been applied. The commonest type of cell junction is the *desmosome*. Desmosomes are found scattered throughout intercellular interfaces where they provide strong points of cohesion between cells and act as anchorage points for the cytoskeleton of each cell. Another widely distributed type of cell junction is the *gap junction* which not only functions as an adherent zone but also permits transfer of information and metabolites between adjacent cells. Between the cells of simple cuboidal and simple columnar epithelia, the intercellular membranes exhibit specialisations called *junctional complexes* which prevent access of luminal contents to the intercellular spaces. Junctional complexes begin immediately below the luminal surface and are made up of three components, one of which is the desmosome; the other two components are called *tight junctions* and *adherent junctions*.

This electron micrograph of a typical junctional complex between two columnar intestinal epithelial cells illustrates tight and adherent junctions and a desmosome; the principal features of these junctions and of a gap junction are shown in the schematic diagram.

(i) Tight junctions: tight junctions **TJ** begin just below the luminal surface and consist of small areas where the outer lamina of opposing plasma membranes are fused with

one another. Between these areas of fusion are areas which are not fused. The tight junction forms a complete circumferential belt around each cell thus sealing the intercellular space from the lumen.

(ii) Adherent junction: adherent junctions **AJ** are found deep to the tight junctions and are areas where the opposing plasma membranes diverge; no structures are evident between the opposing cell membranes. On the cytoplasmic aspect of these junctions, there is a fine mat of filamentous material which merges with the filaments of the cytoskeleton. Like tight junctions, adherent junctions also form a circumferential band around each cell.

(iii) Desmosomes: desmosomes **D** form the third component of junctional complexes but also occur singly at many other intercellular sites. At the desmosome, the opposing plasma membranes are separated by a gap in which many fine, transverse filaments or a dense, longitudinal lamina may be seen. At the cytoplasmic aspect of each plasma membrane there is a closely applied electron-dense layer into which fibrillar elements of the cytoskeleton appear to converge. Desmosomes always appear as the paired structures just described, except at the interface of stratified squamous epithelia and the basement membrane where half desmosomes (*hemi-desmosomes*) can be found.

(iv) Gap junctions: gap junctions are broad areas of closely opposed plasma membranes, but there is no fusion of the plasma membranes and a narrow gap remains. Although this type of junction is a site of intercellular adhesion, gap junctions also permit passage of ions and other molecules between adjacent cells; that is, they are sites of intercellular information exchange.

2. Cell cycle and replication

Introduction

The development of a single, fertilised egg cell to form a complex, multicellular organism involves cellular replication, growth and progressive specialisation for a variety of functions. The mechanism of cellular replication in all but the male and female germ cells is known as *mitosis*. Mitosis or *mitotic division* of a single cell results in the production of two daughter cells, each genetically identical to the parent cell. After the period in which mitosis takes place, the daughter cells enter a period of growth and metabolic activity prior to further mitotic division. The time interval between mitotic divisions, that is the life cycle of an individual cell, is called the *cell cycle*. As development of the fertilised ovum progresses to produce a multicellular embryo, groups of cells and their progeny become increasingly specialised to form tissues each with different specific functions. The process whereby cells become specialised is called *differentiation*. In the fully developed organism, the differentiated cells of some tissues, such as the neurones of the nervous system, lose the ability to undergo mitosis, whereas certain cells of other tissues, such as the epithelial cells lining the gastro-intestinal tract, undergo continuous cycles of mitotic division throughout the lifespan of the organism. Between these extremes, other cells, such as liver cells, do not normally undergo mitosis in the fully developed organism but retain the capacity to undergo mitosis should the need arise.

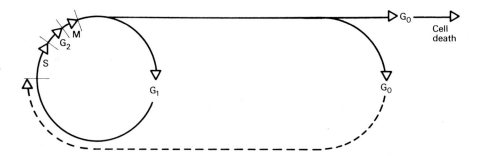

Fig. 2.1 The cell cycle

Historically, only two phases of the cell cycle were recognised; the phase during which mitosis takes place, which in general occurs in a relatively short time, and the phase in which cell division does not take place. This second phase, called *interphase*, usually occupies most of the life cycle of an individual cell. With the development of radio-isotopes it was found that, in cells which undergo mitosis, there is a discrete period during interphase when nuclear DNA is replicated; this phase, described as the *synthesis* or *S phase* of the cell cycle, is completed some time before the onset of mitosis (also called the *M phase*). Thus interphase may be divided into three separate phases. Between the end of the M phase and the beginning of the S phase, the *first gap* or *G_1 phase* occurs; this is usually much longer than the other phases of the cell cycle. During the G_1 phase, cells grow and perform their specialised functions with respect to the tissue as a whole. The interval between the end of the S phase and the beginning of the M phase, the *second gap* or *G_2 phase*, is of relatively short duration and is the period in which cells prepare for mitotic division.

Some cell types progress continuously through the cell cycle in situations where tissue growth or cell turnover is occurring. Cell types which lose the capacity for mitotic division, for example nerve cells, leave the cell cycle after the M phase and enter a protracted functional state

designated as the *G_0 phase*. Some other cell types enter the G_0 phase but retain the capacity to re-enter the cell cycle when suitably stimulated. Some liver cells appear to enter a protracted G_2 phase in which they are fully functional cells despite the presence of more than the usual complement of DNA.

The M phase is usually relatively short and is the period in which DNA, duplicated during the S phase, is equally distributed between the two daughter cells as cell division occurs.

In general, the S, G_2 and M phases of the cell cycle are relatively constant in duration, each taking up to several hours to complete whereas the G_1 phase is highly variable, in some cases lasting for several days or even longer. The G_0 phase may last for the entire lifespan of an individual.

The cell cycle, and hence the rate of cell division, is controlled by both extrinsic and intrinsic factors. Hormones are extrinsic factors which regulate the cell cycles of many cells and thus co-ordinate tissue growth and function. At present, little is known about the intrinsic factors which control the cell cycle. An understanding of all the factors which control the cell cycle is likely to be a prerequisite for elucidation of the primary defect which occurs in conditions of uncontrolled cell division such as cancer.

Mitosis

The process of somatic cell division, or mitosis, occurs in the M phase of the cell cycle and takes approximately 30 to 60 minutes in mammals. Mitosis has two main functions. Firstly, it is the phase in which the chromosomes duplicated in the S phase are distributed equally and identically between the two potential daughter cells; this process is called *karyokinesis*. Secondly, mitosis is the phase in which the dividing cell is cleaved into genetically identical daughter cells by cytoplasmic division or *cytokinesis*. Although karyokinesis is always equal and symmetrical, cytokinesis may, in some situations, result in the formation of two daughter cells with grossly unequal amounts of cytoplasm or cytoplasmic organelles.

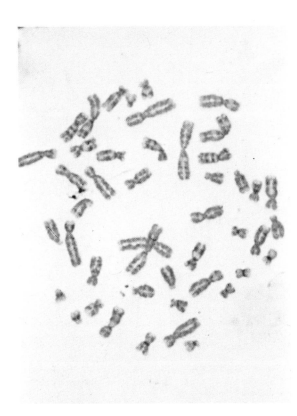

Fig. 2.2 Mitotic chromosomes

(Giemsa × 1200)

In general, the nuclei of all cells contain the same fixed complement of DNA, a quantity called the *genome*. The genome is identical in every cell (except the germ cells and a few odd exceptions) of the same individual. The DNA of the genome is intimately associated with proteins, called nucleo-proteins, and is arranged as a number of discrete strands called *chromosomes*. The cells of each species have a characteristic, fixed number of chromosomes (46 in man) known as *the diploid number*. Chromosomes function in pairs, called *homologous pairs*, the members of each pair having a similar length of DNA and a similar structure.

During interphase, chromosomes exist as an unravelled mass within the nucleus; this arrangement may facilitate gene expression, a process which takes place mainly within the G_1 and G_0 phases of the cell cycle. Histologically, chromosomes are not usually visible within the nucleus of cells in interphase. During the S phase, each chromosome is duplicated and the two identical chromosomes remain attached to each other. At the onset of mitosis, the duplicated chromosomes become tightly coiled and condensed such that they are readily visible with the light microscope. This arrangement of chromosomes during mitosis is merely a mechanism for packaging the duplicated genome which may then be distributed identically and equally between the two daughter cells during mitosis.

This micrograph illustrates the chromosomes of a human cell cultured *in vitro* and arrested at the onset of mitosis; the chromosomes have been treated with the enzyme trypsin, thus revealing a cross-banding pattern along the length of each chromosome. Chromosomes, as seen at mitosis, each consist of a duplicated chromosome, each member of the duplicate being referred to as a *chromatid*. The two so-called chromatids of each chromosome are joined at a point called *the kinetochore* (or *centromere*); this appears as a constriction in each mitotic chromosome.

Each member of a homologous pair of chromosomes is similar in length, kinetochore location and banding pattern. The significance of trypsin-induced chromosomal banding is not understood but the phenomenon provides a useful technique for the identification of chromosomes, especially in the investigation of chromosomal abnormalities.

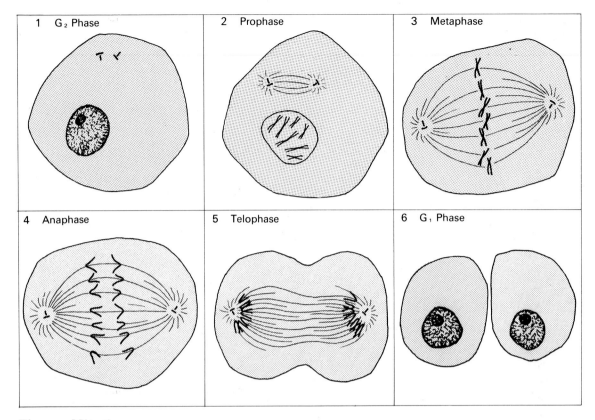

Fig. 2.3 Mitosis

Mitosis is a continuous process which is traditionally divided into four phases: *prophase, metaphase, anaphase* and *telophase*, each stage being readily recognisable with the light microscope. In mammalian cells, both karyokinesis and cytokinesis require the presence of a structure called the *mitotic apparatus*. This structure, which is more fully discussed with Fig. 2.6, consists of longitudinally arranged microtubules which extend between paired organising centres called *centrioles* at the two poles of the dividing cell. Centrioles are discussed further with Fig. 2.6. The mitotic apparatus is visible within the cytoplasm only during the M phase of the cell cycle since it disaggregates shortly after the completion of mitosis.

Prophase: the beginning of this stage of mitosis is defined as the moment when chromosomes first become visible within the nucleus. As prophase continues, the chromosomes become increasingly condensed and shortened and the nucleoli disappear. Dissolution of the nuclear envelope marks the end of prophase. During prophase, the two pairs of centrioles (duplicated earlier in interphase) migrate to opposite poles of the cell. The centrioles remain connected by numerous longitudinal microtubules, collectively forming the so-called *mitotic spindle*; the spindle tubules elongate as the centrioles move apart.

Metaphase: during the second stage of mitosis, the mitotic spindle is completed and the chromosomes become arranged at the equator of the spindle, a region known as the *equatorial* or *metaphase plate*. At this stage the two chromatids of each chromosome are still joined at the kinetochore.

Anaphase: this stage of mitosis is marked by separation of the two chromatids of each chromosome, which then migrate along the spindle to opposite poles of the cell, thus achieving an exact division of the duplicated genetic material. By the end of anaphase, two groups of identical chromosomes (the former chromatids) are clustered at opposite poles of the cell.

Telophase: during the final phase of mitosis, the chromosomes begin to uncoil and to regain their interphase conformation. The nuclear envelope reforms and nucleoli again become apparent. The process of cytokinesis also takes place during telophase; the plane of cytoplasmic division is usually defined by the position of the spindle equator, thus producing two cells of equal size. The plasma membrane around the spindle equator becomes indented to form a circumferential furrow around the cell, the *cleavage furrow*, which progressively constricts the cell until it is cleaved into two daughter cells. In mammalian cells, a ring of microfilaments is present just beneath the surface of the cleavage furrow and it has been suggested that cytokinesis occurs as a result of contraction of this filamentous ring.

In the early G_1 phase, the mitotic spindle disaggregates and in many cell types the single pair of centrioles begins to duplicate in preparation for the next mitotic division. In Fig. 2.4 the four main stages of mitosis are illustrated in actively dividing, primitive blood cells from a smear preparation of bone marrow.

Fig. 2.4 Blood cells in mitosis

(Giemsa ×800)

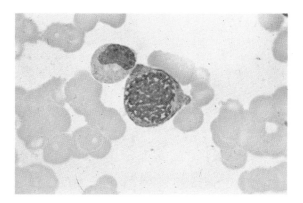

(a) Prophase: this micrograph illustrates a cell in an early stage of prophase. The nucleus consists of a mass of relatively long, discrete chromosomes; nucleoli are not visible. Although the nuclear envelope cannot be resolved by light microscopy, its integrity is implied in this micrograph since the chromosomes have not yet dispersed. Special techniques must be applied before centrioles can be seen with the light microscope.

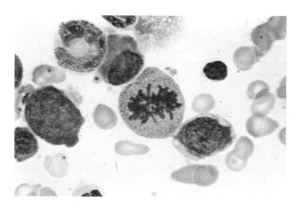

(b) Metaphase: the cell in the centre of the field shows the typical appearance of early metaphase; the chromosomes are more contracted and densely stained and are arranged on the equatorial plate. The mitotic spindle is not seen in this preparation.

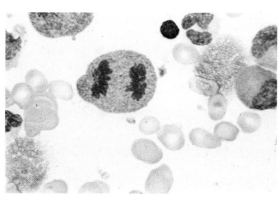

(c) Anaphase: the central cell in this micrograph is in late anaphase. The two groups of identical chromatids have been drawn to opposite poles of the mitotic spindle.

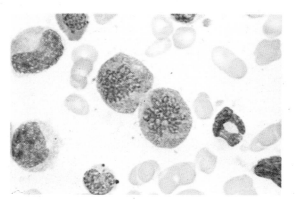

(d) Telophase: in this cell, in late telophase, the process of cytokinesis is almost complete. The two potential daughter cells still remain in contact via a narrow cytoplasmic bridge containing elements of the mitotic spindle. The chromosomes have begun to uncoil and nuclear envelopes are about to form.

Meiosis

In all somatic cells, cell division (mitosis) results in the formation of two daughter cells, each one genetically identical to the mother cell. Somatic cells contain a full complement of chromosomes (the diploid number) which function as homologous pairs as described earlier. The process of sexual reproduction involves the fusion of specialised male and female cells called *gametes* to form a *zygote* which has the diploid number of chromosomes. Each gamete thus contains only half the diploid number of chromosomes; this half complement of chromosomes is known as the *haploid number*.

The production of haploid cells involves a unique form of cell division called *meiosis* which occurs only in the germ cells of the gonads during the formation of gametes; meiotic cell division is thus also called *gametogenesis*. Meiosis involves two cell division processes of which only the first is preceded by duplication of chromosomes.

(i) The first meiotic division results in the formation of two daughter cells; this process differs from mitosis in two important respects:

(a) Whereas in mitosis each chromosome divides at the kinetochore (centromere) liberating two chromatids which migrate to opposite ends of the mitotic spindle, in the first meiotic division there is no such separation of the chromatids but rather one chromosome of each homologous pair migrates to each end of the spindle. Thus at the end of the first meiotic division, each daughter cell contains a half complement of chromosomes, one chromosome being derived from each homologous pair of the mother cell.

(b) During the first meiotic division, and preceding the process described in (a) above, there is an exchange of alleles between the chromosomes of homologous pairs. This exchange, called *chiasma formation*, results in chromosomes with a different genetic constitution from those of the mother cell.

(ii) The second meiotic division merely involves splitting of each chromosome at the kinetochore to liberate chromatids which migrate to opposite poles of the spindle.

Thus, meiotic cell division of a single diploid germ cell gives rise to four haploid gametes. In the male, each of the four gametes undergoes morphological development into a mature spermatozoon whereas in the female, unequal distribution of the cytoplasm during meiosis results in one gamete gaining almost all the cytoplasm from the mother cell, whilst the other three acquire almost no cytoplasm; the large gamete matures to form an *ovum* and the other three, the so-called *polar bodies*, degenerate.

During both the first and second meiotic divisions, the cell passes through stages which have many similar features to prophase, metaphase, anaphase and telophase of mitosis. Unlike mitosis, however, the process of meiotic cell division can be suspended for a considerable length of time. For example, in the development of the human female gamete, the germ cells enter prophase of the first meiotic division during the fifth month of fetal life of the potential mother and then remain suspended until some time after the mother reaches sexual maturity. The first meiotic division is suspended for between twelve and forty-five years.

The primitive germ cells of the male, the *spermatogonia*, are present only in small numbers in the male gonads before sexual maturity. After sexual maturity, spermatogonia multiply continuously by mitosis to provide a supply of cells which then undergo meiosis to form male gametes. In contrast, the germ cells of the female, called *oogonia*, multiply by mitosis only during early fetal development thereby producing a fixed complement of cells with the potential to undergo gametogenesis.

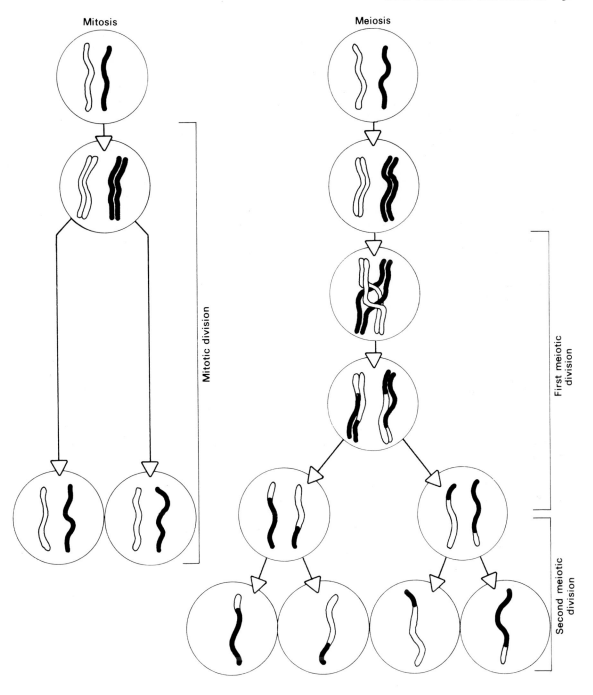

Fig. 2.5 Comparison of mitosis and meiosis

This diagram compares the behaviour of each homologous pair of chromosomes during mitosis and meiosis; note that only one homologous pair is represented here.

The key differences between the two forms of cell division are:

(i) chiasmata formation occurs in meiosis only;

(ii) meiosis involves two sequential cell divisions, the first meiotic cell division resulting in reduction of the chromosome complement to the duplicated haploid state and the second meiotic division resulting in the production of four haploid daughter cells, or gametes.

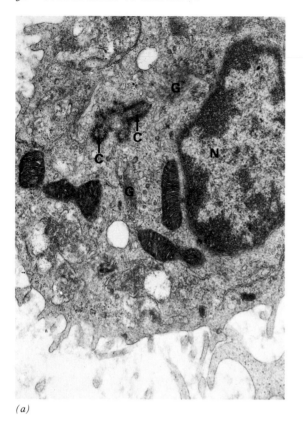

(a)

(b)

Fig. 2.6 Centrosome

(EM (a) ×9200 (b) ×48 000)

The *centrosome* is a zone of cytoplasm usually centrally located in the cell adjacent to the nucleus **N** and often surrounded by the Golgi apparatus **G**. The centrosome, the *cell centre*, contains a pair of centrioles **C** together known as a *diplosome*. Centrioles are structures involved in formation of the mitotic apparatus along which chromosomes migrate during mitosis..Each centriole is a hollow cylinder, closed at one end, and consisting of nine triplets of parallel microtubules; in transverse section, each triplet **T** is seen to consist of an inner microtubule which is circular in cross-section and two further microtubules which are C-shaped in cross-section. Each of the inner microtubules is connected to the outermost microtubule of the adjacent triplet by a fine filament **F**, thus forming a continuous cylinder. The two centrioles of each diplosome are arranged with their long axes at right angles to each other as can be seen in these micrographs; the significance of this arrangement is obscure.

During interphase, and even occasionally during late telophase, diplosomes reduplicate in readiness for the next mitotic division. In prophase, the two pairs of centrioles migrate to opposite poles of the cell but remain connected to each other via the microtubules of the mitotic spindle. It has been suggested that this movement of the centriole pairs is mediated by the spindle microtubules which become progressively elongated by addition of further, preformed subunits of the protein *tubulin* from the cytoplasm. Formerly it was thought that spindle microtubules grew out from the centrioles but it is now believed that centrioles merely act as nucleation centres for microtubule formation.

During metaphase, each chromosome becomes attached to the spindle by the kinetochore; microtubules have been shown to extend from the kinetochore to each pole of the spindle. Although the mechanism by which the chromatids are drawn apart during anaphase is poorly understood, two main theories have emerged. In one theory it is proposed that the pole-to-kinetochore microtubules shorten in length by loss of tubulin subunits at the polar ends of the microtubules; as the microtubules shorten, the chromatids are pulled along towards the poles. In the other main theory, it is suggested that spindle elements form contractile units since one of the contractile proteins of muscle, actin, has been identified biochemically in isolated mitotic spindles. Little is known about the contribution of the mitotic spindle in defining the site of cleavage during cytokinesis; this usually occurs in the plane of the spindle equator.

In addition to their role in mitosis, centrioles also form the basal bodies of cilia and flagella.

Part B   Basic tissue types

Blood
Connective tissue
Epithelium
Muscle
Nervous tissues

3. Blood

Introduction

Blood is a tissue which consists of a variety of cells suspended in a fluid medium called *plasma*. Blood functions principally as a vehicle for the transport of gases, nutrients, metabolic waste products, cells and hormones throughout the body. Thus any sample of blood is composed not only of cells and molecules involved in transport processes but also cells and molecules in the process of being transported.

Plasma is essentially an aqueous solution of inorganic salts which is constantly exchanged with the extracellular fluid medium of all body tissues. Plasma also contains proteins, the *plasma proteins*, of three main types: *albumins*, *globulins* and *fibrinogen*. Collectively, the plasma proteins exert a colloidal osmotic pressure within the circulatory system which helps to regulate the exchange of aqueous solution between plasma and extracellular fluid. The albumins, which constitute the bulk of plasma proteins, bind relatively insoluble metabolites such as fatty acids and thus serve as transport proteins. The globulins are a diverse group of proteins which include the antibodies of the immune system and certain proteins responsible for the transport of lipids and some heavy metal ions. Fibrinogen is a soluble protein which polymerises to form the insoluble protein *fibrin* during blood clotting. In general, the molecular components of plasma cannot be demonstrated by light and electron microscopy.

The cells of blood are of three major functional classes: *red blood cells (erythrocytes)*, *white blood cells (leucocytes)* and *platelets (thrombocytes)*. Erythrocytes are primarily involved in oxygen and carbon dioxide transport, the leucocytes constitute an important part of the defence and immune systems of the body, and platelets are a vital component of the blood clotting mechanism. All these cell types are formed in the bone marrow. Erythrocytes and platelets function entirely within blood vessels whereas leucocytes act mainly outside blood vessels in the tissues. Thus the leucocytes found in circulating blood are merely in transit between their various sites of activity.

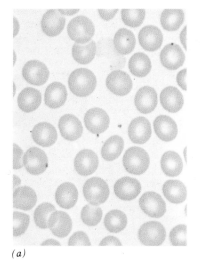
(a)

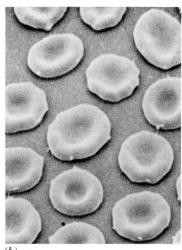
(b)

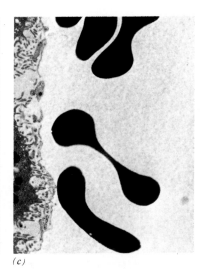
(c)

Fig. 3.1 Red blood cells

(a) Giemsa × 800
(b) Scanning EM × 2400
(c) EM × 5700

Features of red blood cells:

(i) no nucleus (extruded at earlier stage in erythrocyte formation);

(ii) biconcave disc shape greatly enhances surface area relative to cell volume and provides flexibility in passing through small capillaries;

(iii) diameter approximately 7 micrometres;

(iv) contain the oxygen carrying pigment haemoglobin.

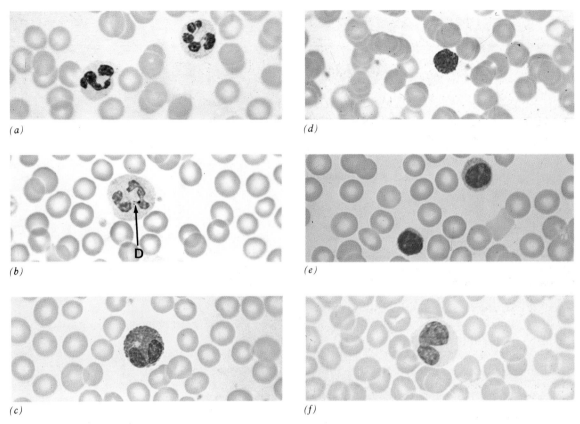

Fig. 3.2 White blood cells

(Giemsa ×800)

(a) Neutrophils: highly lobulated nucleus, neutral staining cytoplasmic granules; highly phagocytic cells which engulf bacteria and damaged tissues; dead and dying polymorphs are known as 'pus cells' and are the major constituent of pus.

(b) Neutrophils with drumstick chromosome: D – drumstick chromosome; represents second X chromosome of nucleus in the female which is condensed and relatively inactive; drumstick chromosome visible in about three per cent of neutrophils of female blood.

(c) Eosinophil: lobulated (usually bilobed) nucleus, large eosinophilic (red stained) cytoplasmic granules; phagocytic, but function not well understood; eosinophils more prolific in allergic states, e.g. asthma and hay fever, and parasitic infestations, e.g. hookworm and bilharzia.

(d) Basophil: lobulated nucleus usually partly obscured by intensely basophilic (blue stained) cytoplasmic granules; function poorly understood but thought to be analogous to mast cells of connective tissue (see Fig. 4.12) which mediate certain allergic states, e.g. asthma and hay fever.

(e) Lymphocytes: spherical nucleus with large nucleo-cytoplasmic ratio; principal cells of the immune system (details given in Fig. 18.1).

(f) Monocyte: largest of the white blood cells; extensive pale-stained cytoplasm and large horseshoe-shaped nucleus; highly phagocytic especially for tissue debris and foreign bodies; analogous to macrophages of connective tissue (see Fig. 4.13).

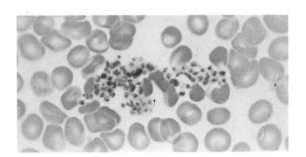

Fig. 3.3 Platelets

(Giemsa ×800)

Small non-nucleated cells derived by 'pinching off' from the cytoplasm of huge cells called megakaryocytes found in bone marrow; platelets perform two functions in stopping bleeding. Firstly in the normal circulation they plug minute defects constantly occurring in the endothelium as a result of normal functional stresses. Secondly, after more major tissue damage, they participate in blood clotting in several ways including aggregation and release of various factors which enhance activation of the clotting cascade.

4. Connective tissue

Introduction

Connective tissue is the term applied to a basic type of tissue of mesodermal origin which provides structural and metabolic support for other tissues and organs throughout the body. Connective tissues carry blood vessels and mediate the exchange of metabolites between tissues and the circulatory system. Rigid forms of connective tissue, particularly cartilage and bone, comprise the major tissues of the skeleton (see Chapter 12). Connective tissue has important metabolic roles such as the storage of fat, as in adipose tissue, whilst connective tissue elements constitute a major part of the body's defence mechanisms against pathogenic micro-organisms. The processes of tissue repair are largely a function of connective tissues. All connective tissues have two major constituents, *cells* and *extracellular material*.

The cells of connective tissue may be divided into three types according to their basic function:

(i) Cells responsible for synthesis and maintenance of the extracellular material. These cells are termed *fibroblasts*.

(ii) Cells responsible for the storage and metabolism of fat. These cells are individually known as *adipocytes* and may collectively form *adipose connective tissue*.

(iii) Cells with defence and immune functions.

Extracellular material is the constituent which mainly determines the physical properties of each type of connective tissue. Extracellular material consists of a matrix of organic material called *ground substance* within which are embedded a variety of *fibres*. Ground substance is an amorphous, transparent material which has the properties of a semi-fluid gel. Tissue fluid is loosely bound to ground substance, thereby forming the medium for passage of materials throughout connective tissues and for the exchange of metabolites with the circulatory system. The molecular composition of ground substance is principally that of long, unbranched chains of large acidic polysaccharides bound to variable amounts of protein. These large molecules are intimately entangled to confer the basic physical properties of connective tissue; the mechanical properties are reinforced by the presence of fibres.

The fibrous components of connective tissue are of three main types: *collagenous, reticular* and *elastic*. These fibres are present in all connective tissues but occur in varying proportions. Classification of the basic connective tissues depends on the predominant fibre type. Collagenous connective tissue is the most common type; the density of collagen fibres varies greatly from loose to dense according to the mechanical supporting function. The regularity and arrangement of collagen fibres also varies according to function. Reticular connective tissue forms a delicate supporting framework for highly cellular organs such as liver, lymph nodes and endocrine glands. Elastic connective tissues contain, as their predominant fibre type, a highly elastic protein called *elastin*, which may be arranged into fibres or discontinuous sheets.

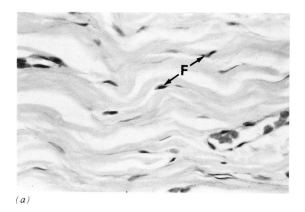

(a)

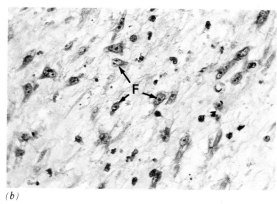

(b)

Fig. 4.1 Fibroblasts

(H & E × 320; (a) mature fibroblasts (b) active fibroblasts)

F – fibroblasts; cells responsible for synthesis and maintenance of extracellular constituents of connective tissue. Active fibroblasts are plump with large nuclei and prominent nucleoli reflecting extensive protein synthesis, e.g. in a healing wound. Mature fibroblasts have contracted, condensed nucleus and cytoplasm is reduced to minute strands extending into the extracellular substance.

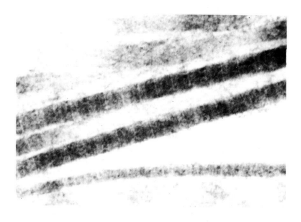

Fig. 4.2 Collagen fibres

(EM × 124000)

Four forms of collagen are recognisable by electron microscopy; this form with prominent cross banding is the type found in common connective tissues.

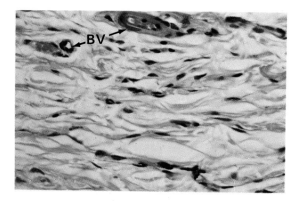

Fig. 4.3 Loose (areolar) connective tissue

(H & E × 320)

Loose, wavy arrangements of collagen fibres (stained pink) with ground substance (unstained) filling the spaces; nuclei are those of fibroblasts. Loose connective tissue is usually found as a supporting tissue for epithelial linings of tubes and ducts or as packing between different tissues and organs; it conveys blood vessels **BV** and nerves, and permits diffusion of metabolites.

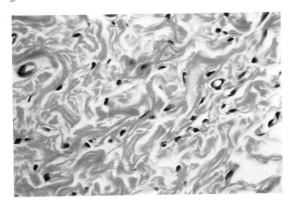

Fig. 4.4 Dense irregular connective tissue
(H & E × 320)

Dense irregular arrangement of collagen fibres with relatively little intervening ground substance; this tissue is tough and resistant and is therefore most commonly seen as supporting tissue for the skin.

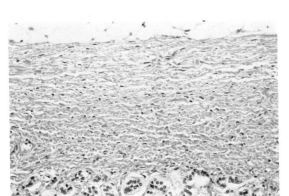

Fig. 4.5 Dense regular connective tissue
(H & E × 128)

Dense collagen arranged in linear fashion; most commonly found forming capsules of organs (in this case the adrenal gland); similar but even more dense regular connective tissue forms tendons, ligaments and joint capsules (see Fig. 12.17).

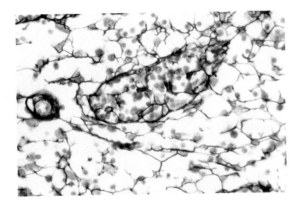

Fig. 4.6 Reticular connective tissue
(Silver method/haematoxylin × 800)

Reticulin fibres are composed of a different form of collagen from that of common connective tissues; although present in all tissues, reticulin is the predominant fibre type in organs such as liver, lymph nodes and endocrine glands where it provides a delicate supporting framework. Reticulin fibres can only be demonstrated by heavy metal impregnation techniques.

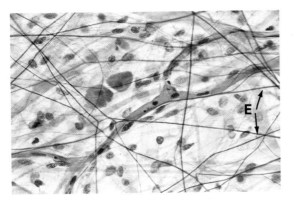

Fig. 4.7 Elastic connective tissue
(Spread preparation; H & E × 320)

Elastin is a different protein from collagen; it has elastic properties and is present to varying degrees in all soft connective tissues. In loose connective tissues, elastin is in the form of branching fibres **E** seen as darkly stained threads in this preparation.

Adipose tissue

Most connective tissues contain cells which are adapted for the storage of fat; these cells are known as adipocytes and may be found in isolation or in clumps throughout loose connective tissue, or may constitute the main cell type as in adipose tissue.

There are two main types of adipose tissue, white and brown:

(i) White adipose tissue: this type of adipose tissue comprises up to 20 per cent of total body weight in normal well nourished male adults and up to 25 per cent in females. It is distributed throughout the body particularly in the deep layers of the skin. In addition to being an important energy store, white adipose tissue acts as a thermal insulator under the skin and functions as a cushion against mechanical forces in such sites as around the kidneys.

(ii) Brown adipose tissue: this highly specialised type of adipose tissue is found in newborn mammals and some hibernating animals, where it plays an important part in body temperature regulation. Only small amounts of brown adipose tissue are found in human adults where its function is thought to contribute little to thermoregulation. Brown adipose tissue is an important site of heat production in newborn humans, in whom heat loss is great largely because of a high body surface area to volume ratio.

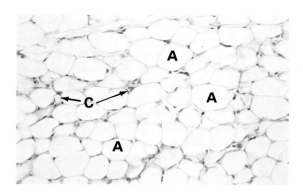

Fig. 4.8 White adipose tissue
(H & E × 128)

A – adipocyte; nucleus compressed and displaced to the periphery of the cell by a single large globule of lipid; lipid is unstained by most histological methods.
C – capillaries; note their minute diameter in relation to that of adipocytes.

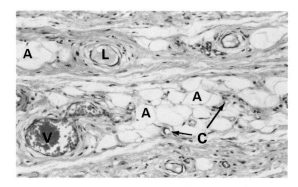

Fig. 4.9 Fibro-fatty connective tissue
(H & E × 128)

A – adipocytes; typical appearance when scattered in loose connective tissue
V – venule
C – capillaries
L – lymphatics

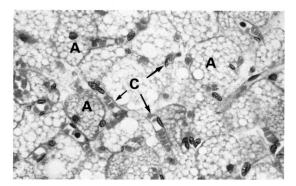

Fig. 4.10 Brown adipose tissue
(H & E × 320)

A – brown adipocytes; in contrast to white adipose tissue, brown adipocytes contain numerous small lipid droplets. Nuclei are plump and not displaced to the periphery of the cell.
C – capillaries; note the extensive capillary network.

The defence cells of connective tissue

The basic connective tissues not only contain cells responsible for synthesis, maintenance and metabolic activity, but also contain a variety of cells with defence and immune functions. Traditionally, these cells have been divided into two categories: fixed (intrinsic) cells and wandering (extrinsic) cells. The fixed category included *tissue macrophages* and *mast cells*. Tissue macrophages are now generally believed to be derived from circulating monocytes (see Chapter 3) which have become at least temporarily resident in connective tissues. Mast cells are functionally analogous to basophils (see Chapter 3) but there are structural differences which suggest that mast cells are not merely basophils resident in connective tissues. The wandering category of defence and immune cells includes all the remaining members of the white blood cell series (see Chapter 3). Although leucocytes are usually considered as a constituent of blood, their principal site of activity is outside the blood circulation, particularly within loose connective tissues. Leucocytes are normally found only in relatively small numbers within connective tissues but in response to inflammation and other disease processes their numbers increase greatly. The connective tissues of those regions of the body which are subject to the constant threat of pathogenic invasion, such as the gastro-intestinal and respiratory tracts, contain a large population of leucocytes, even in the absence of overt disease.

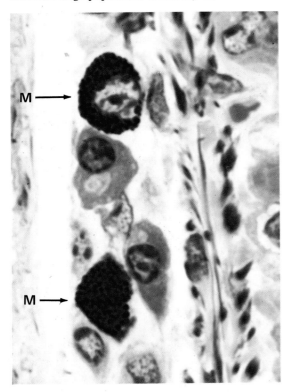

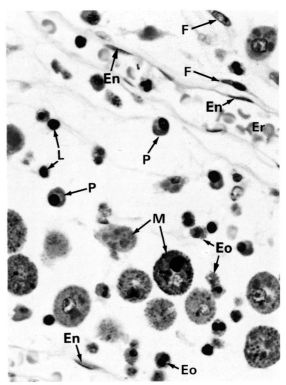

Fig. 4.11 Mast cells

(Toluidine blue × 1200)

M – mast cells; cytoplasm contains large, strongly basophilic granules (which turn red with this staining method); granules contain various vasoactive substances including histamine which increases capillary permeability and causes dilatation of small vessels; histamine release is responsible for some important features of allergic states such as hay fever and asthma.

Fig. 4.12 Leucocytes in loose connective tissue

(H & E ×640)

Eo – eosinophils (see Fig. 3.2(c))
L – lymphocytes (see Fig. 3.2(e))
M – macrophages (see Fig. 3.2(f)); responsible for phagocytosis of tissue debris and foreign bodies; appearance reflects degree of phagocytic activity; here the macrophages are swollen with numerous brown-stained phagosomes (see Fig. 3.1)
P – plasma cells; form of lymphocytes responsible for secretion of antibodies (see Chapter 18)
F – fibroblasts
En – capillary endothelial cells
Er – erythrocytes

5. Epithelium

Introduction

The epithelia are a diverse group of tissues which, with rare exceptions, line all body surfaces, cavities and tubes. Epithelia thus function as interfaces between biological compartments. Epithelial interfaces are involved in a wide range of activities such as absorption, secretion and protection and all these major functions may be exhibited at a single epithelial surface. For example, the epithelial lining of the small intestine is primarily involved in absorption of the products of digestion, but the epithelium also protects itself from noxious intestinal contents by the secretion of a surface coating of mucus.

Surface epithelia consist of one or more layers of cells separated by a minute quantity of intercellular material and closely bound to one another by a variety of specialisations of the cell membrane (see Fig. 1.19). All epithelia are supported by a *basement membrane* of variable thickness. Basement membranes separate epithelia from underlying connective tissues and are never penetrated by blood vessels; epithelia are thus dependent on the diffusion of oxygen and metabolites from underlying tissues. Basement membranes consist of a condensation of glycoprotein ground substance reinforced by reticular fibres which merge with those of the underlying connective tissue.

Epithelia are classified according to three morphological characteristics:

(i) The number of cell layers: a single layer of epithelial cells is termed *simple epithelium*, whereas epithelia composed of more than one layer are termed *stratified epithelia*.

(ii) The shape of the component cells when seen in sections taken at right angles to the epithelial surface: in stratified epithelia the shape of the outermost layer of cells determines the descriptive classification. Cellular outlines are often difficult to distinguish, but the shape of epithelial cells is usually reflected in the shape of their nuclei.

(iii) The presence of surface specialisations such as cilia and keratin: an example is the epithelial surface of skin which is classified as 'stratified squamous keratinising epithelium' since it consists of many layers of cells, the surface cells of which are flattened (squamous) in shape and covered by an outer layer of the proteinaceous material, keratin (see Fig. 14.3).

Epithelia may be derived from ectoderm, mesoderm or endoderm although in the past it was thought that true epithelia were only of ectodermal or endodermal origin; two types of epithelia derived from mesoderm, the lining of blood and lymphatic vessels and the linings of the serous body cavities, were not considered to be epithelia and were termed *endothelium* and *mesothelium* respectively. By both morphological and functional criteria, such distinction has little practical value, nevertheless, the terms endothelium and mesothelium are still used to describe these types of epithelium.

Epithelium which is primarily involved in secretion is often arranged into structures called *glands*. Glands are merely invaginations of epithelial surfaces which are formed during embryonic development by proliferation of epithelium into the underlying connective tissues. Those glands which maintain their continuity with the epithelial surface via a duct are called *exocrine glands* and secrete on to the free surface. In some cases, the duct degenerates during development to leave isolated islands of epithelial secretory tissue deep within other tissues. These glands, known as *endocrine* or *ductless glands*, secrete directly into the bloodstream and their secretions are known as hormones; in addition, some endocrine glands develop by migration of epithelial cells into connective tissues, without the formation of a duct.

Simple epithelia

Simple epithelia are defined as surface epithelia consisting of a single layer of cells. Simple epithelia are almost always found on absorptive or secretory surfaces; they provide little protection against mechanical abrasion and thus are almost never found on surfaces subject to such stresses. The cells comprising simple epithelia range in shape from extremely flattened to tall columnar, depending on their function. For example, flattened simple epithelia present little barrier to passive diffusion and are therefore found in sites such as the lung alveoli and the lining of blood vessels. In contrast, highly active epithelial cells, such as the cells lining the small intestine, are generally tall since they must accommodate the appropriate organelles. Simple epithelia may exhibit a variety of surface specialisations, such as microvilli and cilia, which facilitate their specific surface functions.

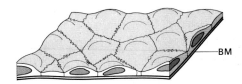

Fig. 5.1 Simple squamous epithelium

Flattened, irregularly shaped cells arranged like 'crazy paving'; permits passive diffusion of gases, e.g. lung alveoli, and fluids, e.g. capillary walls and lining of pleural, pericardial and peritoneal cavities.

BM – basement membrane

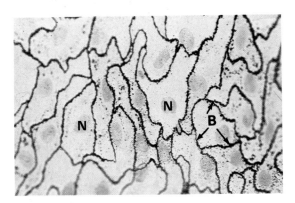

Fig. 5.2 Simple squamous epithelium: lining of peritoneal cavity

(Spread preparation: silver method × 320)

N – nuclei of simple squamous cells
B – intercellular boundaries

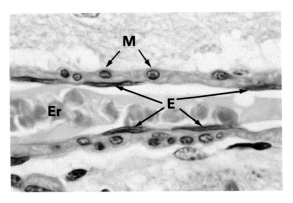

Fig. 5.3 Simple squamous epithelium: small blood vessel

(H & E × 800)

E – nuclei of simple squamous epithelial cells (endothelium)
M – nuclei of smooth muscle cells of blood vessel wall
Er – erythrocytes

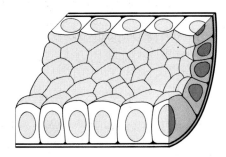

Fig. 5.4 Simple cuboidal epithelium

Cells appear cuboid in cross section although actually have polyhedral shape on luminal surface; may be involved in secretory or absorptive functions and usually form lining of small tubules or ducts, e.g. kidney, salivary glands, pancreas.

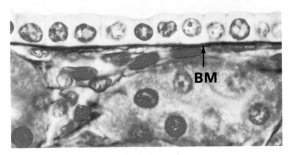

Fig. 5.5 Simple cuboidal epithelium: kidney collecting tubule

(Azan × 800)

BM – basement membrane

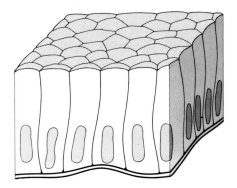

Fig. 5.6 Simple columnar epithelium

Cells appear tall and columnar in cross section; height of cells variable; usually found at highly absorptive surfaces, e.g. small intestine.

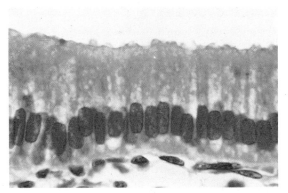

Fig. 5.7 Simple columnar epithelium: gall bladder

(H & E ×800)

The cells shown in this micrograph are from the inner lining of the gall bladder; in this site they are involved in the reabsorption of water from bile, thus concentrating the bile solution.

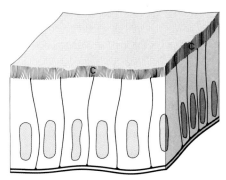

Fig. 5.8 Simple columnar ciliated epithelium

C – cilia

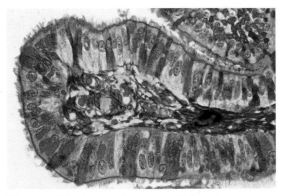

Fig. 5.9 Simple columnar ciliated epithelium: oviduct

(Azan ×320)

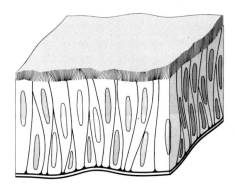

Fig. 5.10 Pseudostratified columnar ciliated epithelium

In pseudostratified epithelium there appears to be more than one layer of cells but in fact all cells rest on the basement membrane.

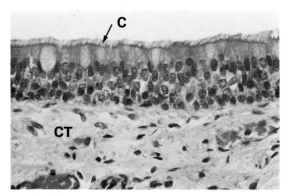

Fig. 5.11 Pseudostratified columnar ciliated epithelium: trachea

(H & E ×320)

C – cilia
CT – supporting loose connective tissue

Stratified epithelia

Stratified epithelia are defined as epithelia consisting of two or more layers of cells. In contrast to simple epithelia, stratified epithelia primarily have a protective function and the degree and nature of the stratification is related to the kinds of physical stresses to which the surface is exposed. In general, stratified epithelia are poorly suited for the functions of absorption and secretion by virtue of their thickness, although some stratified surfaces are moderately permeable to water and other small molecules. The classification of the various stratified epithelia usually relates to the structure of the surface layer since cells of the basal layer are, in general, cuboidal in shape.

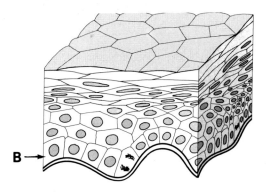

Fig. 5.12 Stratified squamous epithelium

B – basal layer; site of mitosis; cells progressively pushed towards surface where they are continuously shed

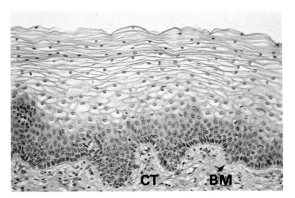

Fig. 5.13 Stratified squamous epithelium: vagina

(H & E × 128)

BM – basement membrane
CT – supporting connective tissue

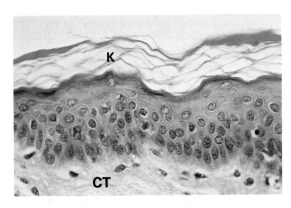

Fig. 5.14 Stratified squamous keratinising epithelium: skin

(H & E × 320)

K – keratin; tough proteinaceous material and remnants of degenerate surface cells
CT – supporting connective tissue

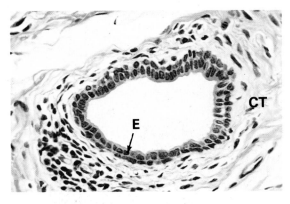

Fig. 5.15 Stratified cuboidal epithelium: salivary gland duct

(H & E × 320)

E – stratified cuboidal epithelium; usually only two or three cell layers thick
CT – supporting connective tissue

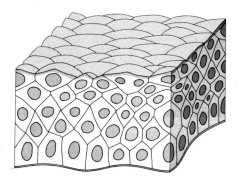

Fig. 5.16 Transitional epithelium

Exclusively confined to the urinary system in mammals; basal cells roughly cuboidal, intermediate cells polygonal, surface cells large and rounded and sometimes binucleate; nuclei of surface cells have prominent nucleoli; transitional epithelium can accommodate much stretching, and appearance varies greatly according to degree of stretch.

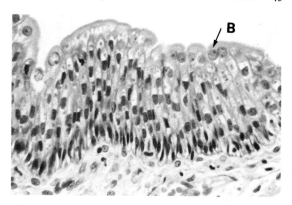

Fig. 5.17 Transitional epithelium: urinary bladder

(H & E × 320)

B – binucleate surface cell

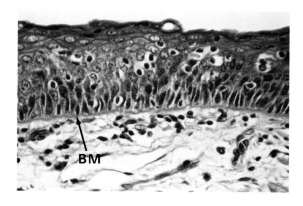

Fig. 5.18 Basement membrane

(PAS × 320)

BM – basement membrane; often difficult to identify with routine staining methods but always present between epithelium and supporting connective tissue; composed of glycoproteins which are well demonstrated by this technique which stains them red.

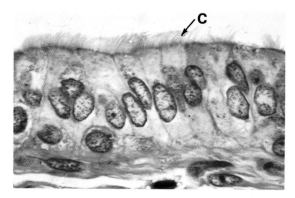

Fig. 5.19 Cilia

(Bronchiole: toluidine blue × 800)

C – cilia; may be 7–10 micrometres in length; up to 300 cilia per cell; beat in a wave-like fashion.

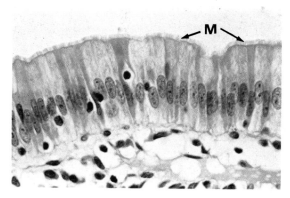

Fig. 5.20 Microvilli

(Small intestine: H & E × 320)

M – microvilli; minute fingerlike projections of surface plasma membrane; much shorter and more delicate in comparison with cilia; up to 3000 microvilli per cell giving appearance of 'brush' or 'striated' border.

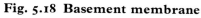

Glands

Exocrine glands are composed of epithelial cells which are specialised for secretion; they may be classified according to two major characteristics:

(i) The morphology of the gland: exocrine glands may be broadly divided into simple and compound glands. *Simple glands* are defined as those with a single, unbranched duct. The secretory portions of simple glands have two main forms, tubular or acinar, which may be coiled and/or branched. *Compound glands* have a branched duct system. The secretory portions of compound glands have similar morphological forms to those of the simple glands with the exception that both tubular and acinar forms may be found together draining into the same duct system. The morphology of the various exocrine gland types is summarised in Fig. 5.21 and examples are shown in Figs. 5.22 to 5.29.

(ii) The means of discharge of secretory products from the cells:

(a) *merocrine*. Merocrine secretion is an alternative name applied to the process of exocytosis (see Chapter 1) and is the most common form of secretion. It is also known as *eccrine* secretion.

(b) *apocrine*. Apocrine secretion involves the discharge of free, unbroken, membrane-bound vesicles containing secretory products and is an unusual means of secretion of lipid products in such glands as the breasts and some sweat glands.

(c) *holocrine*. This is another unusual form of secretion which involves the discharge of whole secretory cells with subsequent disintegration of the cells to release the secretory product. Holocrine secretion occurs principally in sebaceous glands.

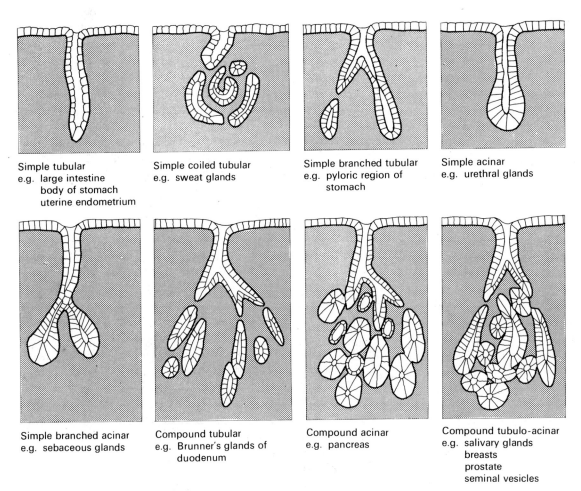

Simple tubular
e.g. large intestine
    body of stomach
    uterine endometrium

Simple coiled tubular
e.g. sweat glands

Simple branched tubular
e.g. pyloric region of
    stomach

Simple acinar
e.g. urethral glands

Simple branched acinar
e.g. sebaceous glands

Compound tubular
e.g. Brunner's glands of
    duodenum

Compound acinar
e.g. pancreas

Compound tubulo-acinar
e.g. salivary glands
    breasts
    prostate
    seminal vesicles

Fig. 5.21 Exocrine gland types

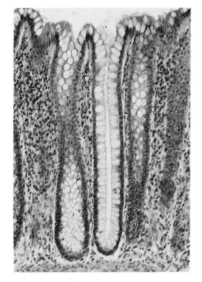

Fig. 5.22 Simple tubular glands

(Large intestine: H & E ×50)

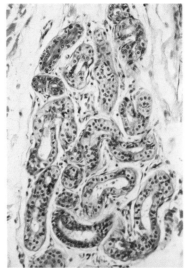

Fig. 5.23 Simple coiled tubular gland

(Sweat gland: H & E ×80)

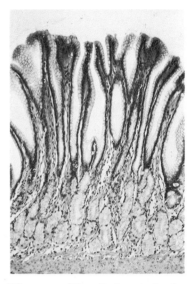

Fig. 5.24 Simple branched tubular glands

(Pyloric stomach: H & E ×50)

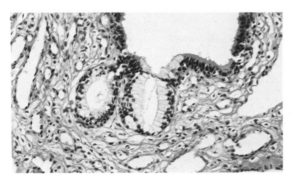

Fig. 5.25 Simple acinar glands

(Penile urethra: H & E ×128)

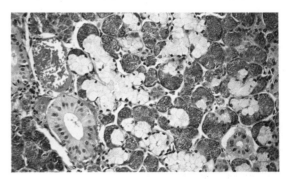

Fig. 5.26 Compound tubulo-acinar gland

(Salivary gland: H & E ×128)

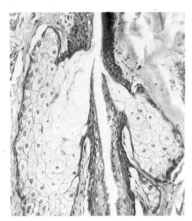

Fig. 5.27 Simple branched acinar gland

(Sebaceous gland: Masson's trichrome ×80)

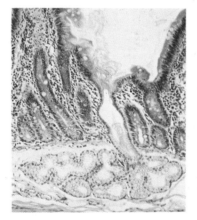

Fig. 5.28 Compound tubular gland

(Brunner's gland of duodenum: H & E ×20)

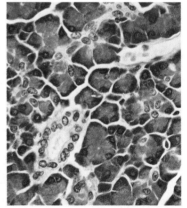

Fig. 5.29 Compound acinar gland

(Pancreas: chrome alum haematoxylin phloxine ×320)

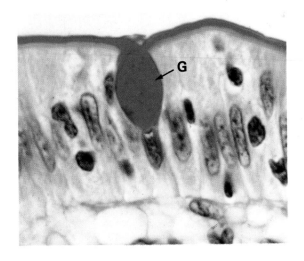

Fig. 5.30 Goblet cell
(PAS/haematoxylin ×800)

G – goblet cell; modified columnar epithelial cell specialised for synthesis of mucus; scattered in epithelial linings of gastro-intestinal and respiratory tracts; mucus is predominantly composed of mucopolysaccharides which stain magenta with this technique.

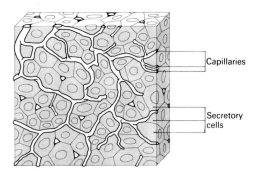

Fig. 5.31 Endocrine gland

Ductless gland which secretes hormones which are absorbed directly into the circulation; rich network of capillaries in all endocrine glands.

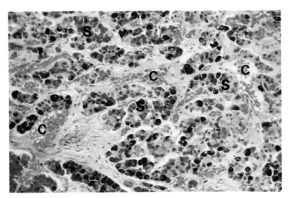

Fig. 5.32 Endocrine gland
(Anterior pituitary: isamine blue/eosin ×128)

S – secretory cells (of various different types and staining characteristics in the pituitary)
C – capillaries

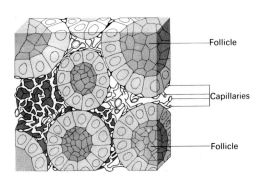

Fig. 5.33 Follicular endocrine gland

The thyroid is an unusual type of endocrine gland which stores hormone in extracellular sites prior to secretion; secretory cells form spherical follicles surrounding hormone which is stored by conjugation with glycoprotein; hormone must be reabsorbed by follicular cells before secretion.

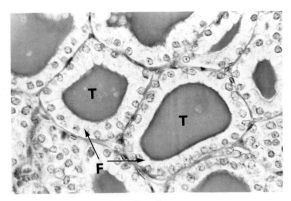

Fig. 5.34 Thyroid gland
(PAS/haematoxylin ×320)

F – follicular cells
T – thyroglobulin, storage form of thyroid hormone

6. Muscle

Introduction

Contractility is an inherent property of all cells which is necessary for the performance of basic functions involving movement such as phagocytosis and cell division, and more specialised functions such as motility as in white blood cells. In multicellular organisms some cells are specialised to enable movement of tissues or organs. These cells may function as single contractile units, such as the myoepithelial cells surrounding the acini of some exocrine glands, or may be aggregated to form muscles for the movement of larger structures. Recent evidence, partly based on the study of the contractile mechanisms of some unicellular organisms, suggests that there is an homologous contractile mechanism in all cells. This mechanism consists of fibrillar proteins arranged in an organised manner in the cytoplasm, and linked by intermolecular bonds. Contraction results from the rearrangement of the intermolecular bonds with the utilisation of chemical energy.

There are three types of muscle tissue:

(i) Skeletal muscle: this is responsible for the movement of the skeleton and organs such as the globe of the eye and the tongue. Skeletal muscle is often referred to as *voluntary muscle* since it may be controlled voluntarily. The arrangement of the contractile proteins gives rise to the appearance of prominent cross-striations in some histological preparations and hence the name *striated muscle* is often applied to skeletal muscle.

(ii) Visceral muscle: this type of muscle forms the muscular component of diverse visceral structures, such as blood vessels, the gastro-intestinal tract, the uterus and the urinary bladder. Since visceral muscle is under inherent, autonomic and hormonal control it is described as *involuntary muscle*. As the arrangement of contractile proteins does not give the histological appearance of cross-striations, the name *smooth muscle* is commonly applied.

(iii) Cardiac muscle: cardiac muscle has many structural and functional characteristics intermediate between those of skeletal and visceral muscle; these provide for the continuous, rhythmic contractility of the heart. Although striated in appearance, cardiac muscle is readily distinguishable from skeletal muscle.

The highly specialised functions of the cytoplasmic organelles of muscle cells has led to the use of a special terminology: plasma membrane or plasmalemma=*sarcolemma*; cytoplasm=*sarcoplasm*; endoplasmic reticulum=*sarcoplasmic reticulum*; mitochondria=*sarcosomes*.

Fig. 6.1 Skeletal muscle

M – muscle fibres (cells); arranged in bundles, individual fibres separated by extremely delicate connective tissue containing small capillaries; bundles separated by more dense connective tissue containing larger vessels; whole muscle mass invested in very dense connective tissue.
C – connective tissue
B – blood vessels

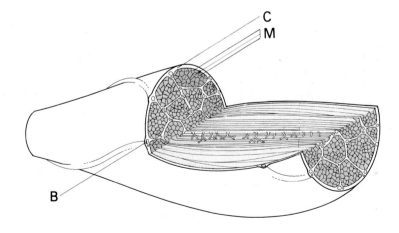

Fig. 6.2 Skeletal muscle

(Tongue: Masson's trichrome ×198)

TS – muscle bundles in transverse section
LS – muscle bundles in longitudinal and oblique section
CT – loose connective tissue containing capillaries and nerves (collagen stains blue with this technique)

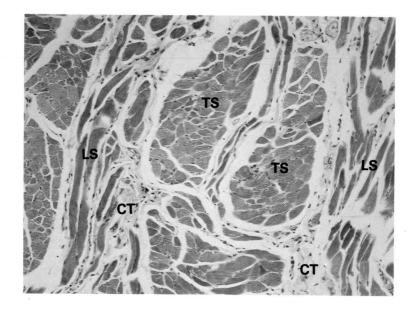

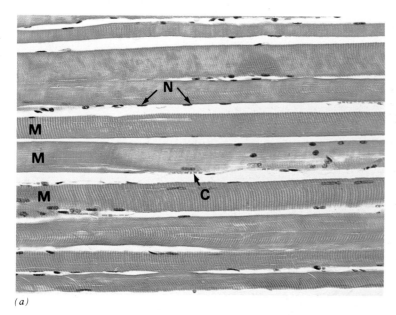

(a)

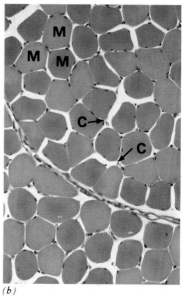

(b)

Fig. 6.3 Skeletal muscle

(a) LS (b) TS: H & E ×300

M – muscle fibres; extremely long, cylindrical shape; cross striations seen in longitudinal section
N – nuclei; skeletal muscle cells are multinucleate and nuclei are located immediately beneath the plasma membrane
C – capillaries

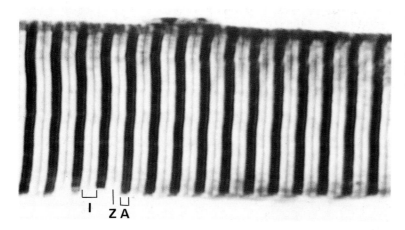

Fig. 6.4 Skeletal muscle

(LS: Heidenhain's haematoxylin × 1200)

I – I band
Z – Z line
A – A band

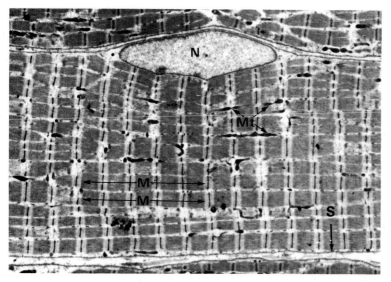

Fig. 6.5 Skeletal muscle

(LS: EM × 2860)

M – myofibrils; made up of sarcomeres arranged end-to-end; myofibrils are unbranched and extend the whole length of the muscle fibre; note that sarcomeres of adjacent myofibrils are in register.
Mt – mitochondria; situated between myofibrils
N – nucleus of muscle fibre
S – sarcolemma (plasma membrane)

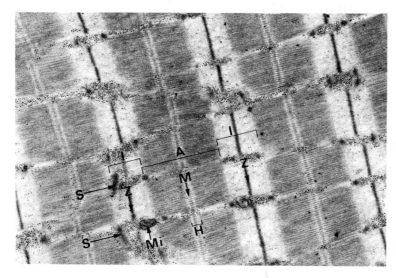

Fig. 6.6 Skeletal muscle: sarcomeres

(EM × 18 700)

I – I band
A – A band
H – H band
Z – Z line
M – M line
Mi – mitochondrion
S – sarcoplasmic reticulum; system of tubules which conducts contractile stimuli deep into muscle cell.

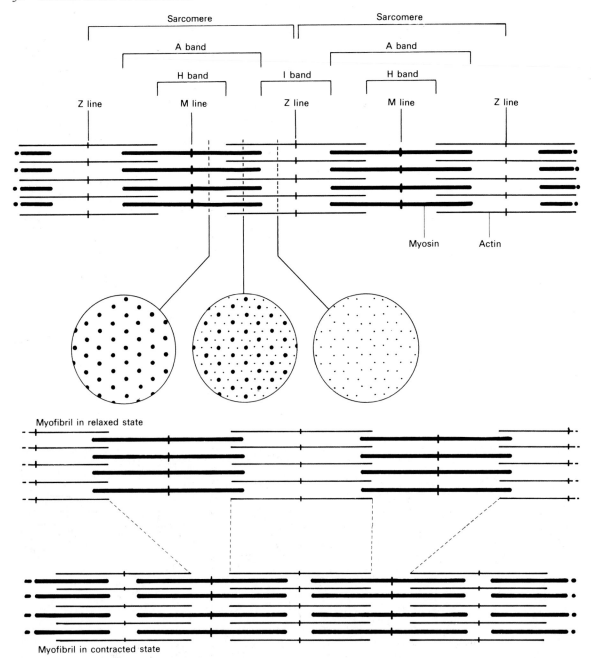

Fig. 6.7 Arrangement of myofilaments in the sarcomere: sliding filament theory of muscular contraction

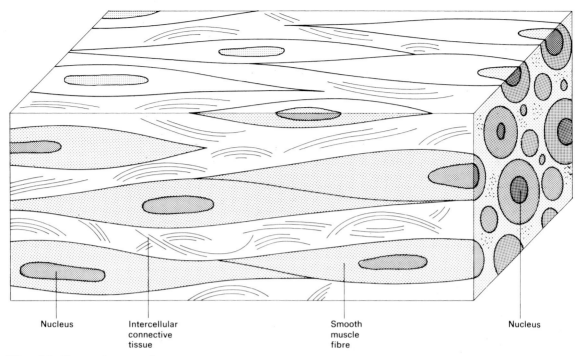

Nucleus Intercellular connective tissue Smooth muscle fibre Nucleus

Fig. 6.8 Smooth muscle

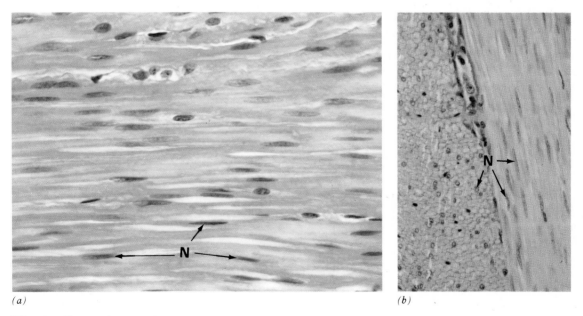

(a)   *(b)*

Fig. 6.9 Smooth muscle

(a) LS: H & E × 480
(b) LS & TS: PAS/iron haematoxylin/orange G × 320
N – smooth muscle nuclei (Smooth muscle cytoplasm
stains pink in (a) and yellow in (b); cell membranes cannot
be distinguished.)

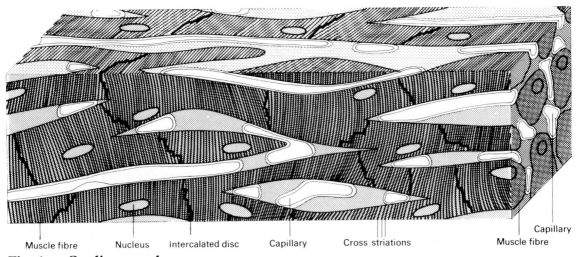

Muscle fibre   Nucleus   Intercalated disc   Capillary   Cross striations

Capillary
Muscle fibre

Fig. 6.10 Cardiac muscle

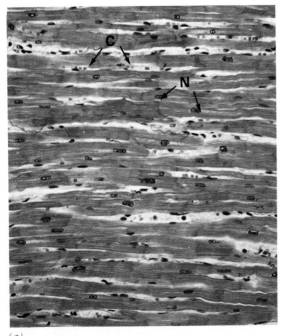

(a)

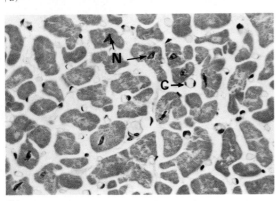

(b)

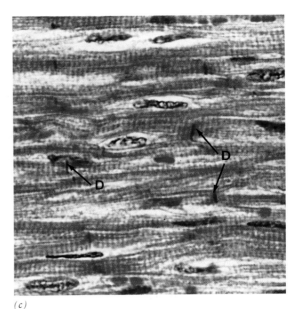

(c)

Fig. 6.11 Cardiac muscle

(a) LS: H & E × 198
(b) TS: H & E × 320
(c) LS: Masson's trichrome × 480

N – cardiac muscle nuclei; centrally located
C – capillaries; cardiac muscle has a very rich vascular supply
D – intercalated discs; specialised low resistance junction between cardiac muscle cells which permits rapid spread of contractile impulses.

7. Nervous tissues

Introduction

The function of the nervous system is to receive stimuli from both the internal and external environments; these are then analysed and integrated to produce appropriate, co-ordinated responses in various effector organs. The nervous system is composed of an intercommunicating network of specialised cells called *neurones* which constitute most sensory receptors, the conducting pathways, and the sites of integration and analysis. The functions of the nervous system depend on a fundamental property of neurones called *excitability*. Like all cells, the resting neurone maintains an ionic gradient across its plasma membrane thereby creating an electrical potential. Excitability involves a change in membrane permeability in response to appropriate stimuli such that the ionic gradient is reversed and the plasma membrane becomes *depolarised*; a wave of depolarisation, known as an *action potential*, then spreads along the plasma membrane; this is followed by the process of *repolarisation* in which the membrane rapidly re-establishes its resting potential. At *synapses*, the sites of intercommunication between adjacent neurones, depolarisation of one neurone causes it to release chemical transmitter substances, *neurotransmitters*, which initiate an action potential in the adjacent neurone. Within the nervous system, neurones are arranged to form pathways for the conduction of action potentials from receptors to effector organs via integrating neurones. Neurotransmitters not only mediate neurone-to-neurone transmission but also act as chemical intermediates between the nervous system and effector organs which also exhibit the property of excitability. The effector organs of voluntary nervous pathways are generally skeletal muscle, and those of involuntary pathways are usually smooth muscle, cardiac muscle and muscle-like epithelial cells (myoepithelial cells) within some exocrine glands.

The nervous system is divided anatomically into the *central nervous system* (CNS) comprising the brain and spinal cord, and the *peripheral nervous system* (PNS) which constitutes all nervous tissue outside the CNS. Functionally, the nervous system is divided into the *somatic nervous system* which is involved in voluntary functions, and the *autonomic nervous system* which exerts control over many involuntary functions. Histologically, however, the entire nervous system merely consists of variations in the arrangement of neurones and their supporting tissues.

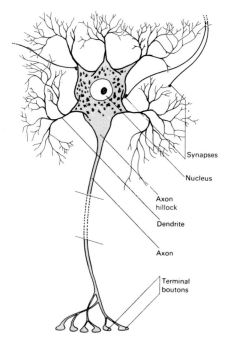

Fig. 7.1 Neurone structure

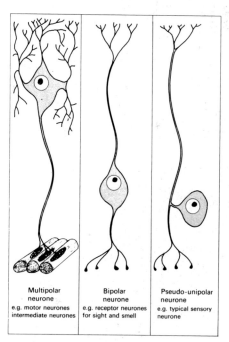

Fig. 7.2 Basic neurone types

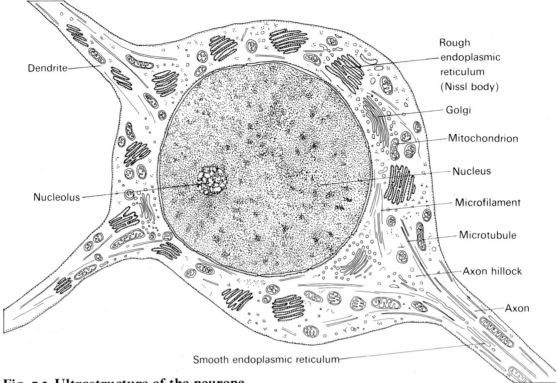

Dendrite

Rough endoplasmic reticulum (Nissl body)

Golgi

Mitochondrion

Nucleus

Microfilament

Microtubule

Axon hillock

Axon

Nucleolus

Smooth endoplasmic reticulum

Fig. 7.3 Ultrastructure of the neurone

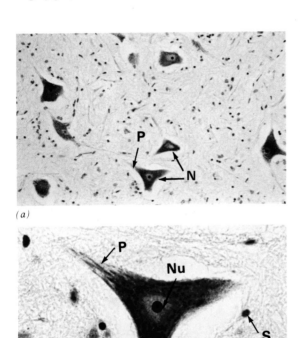

(a)

(b)

Fig. 7.4 Neurones: grey matter
(Nissl method: (a) ×128 (b) ×800)

N – neurone cell bodies
Nu – nucleolus; the nucleus is less well defined
P – neuronal processes, either dendrites or axons
S – nuclei of neurone support cells of various types

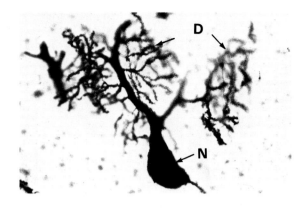

Fig. 7.5 Neurone
(Purkinje cell of cerebellum: Golgi-Cox method × 320)

N – neurone cell body
D – dendritic tree

Myelinated and non-myelinated nerve fibres

In the peripheral nervous system, all axons are enveloped by specialised cells called *Schwann cells* which provide both structural and metabolic support. In general, small diameter axons, for example those of the autonomic nervous system and small pain fibres, are simply enveloped by the cytoplasm of Schwann cells; these nerve fibres are said to be *non-myelinated*. Large-diameter fibres are wrapped by a variable number of concentric layers of the Schwann cell plasma membrane forming the so-called *myelin sheath*; such nerve fibres are said to be *myelinated*. Within the central nervous system, myelination is similar to that in the peripheral nervous system except that the myelin sheaths are formed by cells called *oligodendrocytes*. All non-myelinated fibres in the CNS have no specific cellular support but are indirectly supported by the mass of surrounding tissue.

In all nerve fibres, the rate of conduction of action potentials is proportional to the diameter of the axon; myelination greatly increases axon conduction velocity compared with a non-myelinated fibre of the same diameter.

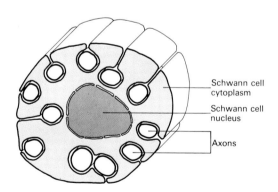

Schwann cell cytoplasm

Schwann cell nucleus

Axons

Fig. 7.6 Non-myelinated nerve fibres

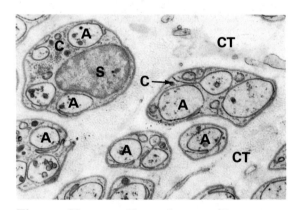

Fig. 7.7 Non-myelinated nerve fibres
(EM × 9450)

A – axons
S – Schwann cell nucleus
C – Schwann cell cytoplasm
CT – delicate supporting tissue

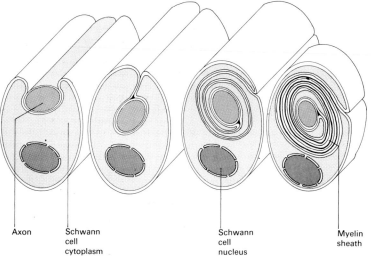

Fig. 7.8 Myelin sheath formation in the peripheral nervous system

Axon

Schwann cell cytoplasm

Schwann cell nucleus

Myelin sheath

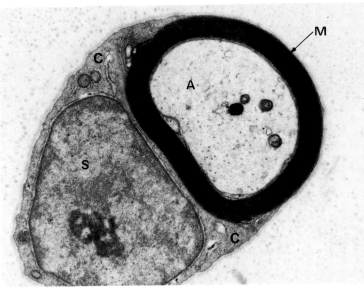

(a)

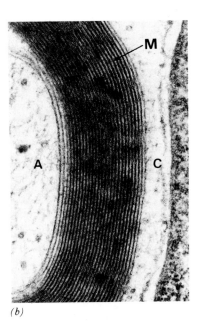

(b)

Fig. 7.9 Myelinated nerve fibre

(EM (a) × 17 000 (b) × 75 250)

S – Schwann cell nucleus   **A** – axon
C – Schwann cell cytoplasm   **M** – myelin sheath

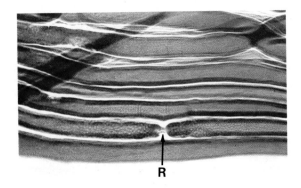

R

Fig. 7.10 Node of Ranvier

(Teased preparation: Sudan black × 320)

R – node of Ranvier; represents gap between portions of myelin sheath provided by different Schwann cells; nerve impulse jumps from node to node thus greatly increasing speed of conduction.

Synapses and neuromuscular junctions

Synapses are highly specialised, intercellular junctions which link the neurones of each nervous pathway, and which link neurones and their effector cells such as muscle fibres; where neurones synapse with skeletal muscle they are referred to as *neuromuscular junctions* or *motor end plates*. Individual neurones intercommunicate via a widely variable number of synapses depending on their location within the nervous system. Classically, the axon of one neurone synapses with the dendrite of another neurone, but axons may synapse with the cell bodies or axons of other neurones; dendrite-to-dendrite and cell body-to-cell body synapses have also been described. For a given synapse, the conduction of an impulse is always in one direction only, but the response may be either excitatory or inhibitory depending on the specific nature of the synapse and its location within the nervous system.

The mechanism of conduction of the nerve impulse is thought to involve the release from one neurone of a chemical transmitter substance, or neurotransmitter, which then diffuses across a narrow intercellular space to induce excitation or inhibition in the other neurone or effector cell of that synapse. Neurotransmitters mediate their effects by interacting with specific receptors incorporated in the opposing plasma membrane.

The chemical nature of neurotransmitters and the morphology of synapses, is highly variable in different parts of the nervous system, but the principles of synaptic transmission and the basic structure of synapses is the same throughout the nervous system.

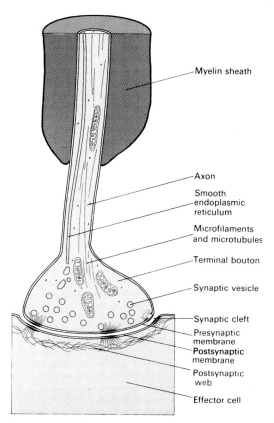

Myelin sheath

Axon

Smooth endoplasmic reticulum

Microfilaments and microtubules

Terminal bouton

Synaptic vesicle

Synaptic cleft

Presynaptic membrane

Postsynaptic membrane

Postsynaptic web

Effector cell

Fig. 7.11 Structure of synapse

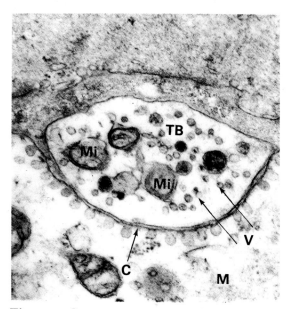

Fig. 7.12 Synapse
(EM × 45 000)

TB – terminal bouton
M – effector muscle cell
Mi – mitochondria in terminal bouton
V – synaptic vesicles
C – synaptic cleft

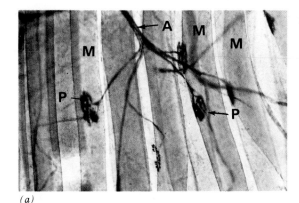

(a)

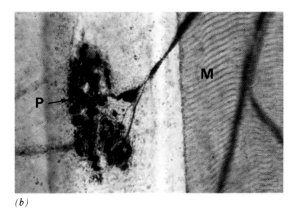

(b)

Fig. 7.13 Motor end plates
*(Teased preparations: gold impregnation method (a) × 320
(b) ×800)*

P – motor end plates; these are neuromuscular junctions
with structure similar to synapse shown in Fig. 7.11
A – axon of motor neurone; note branching to supply
several motor end plates
M – skeletal muscle fibres (effector cells)

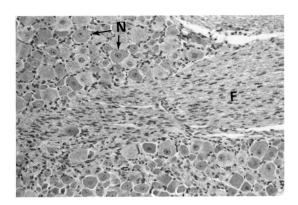

Fig. 7.14 Spinal (dorsal root) ganglion
(H & E × 128)

N – nerve cell bodies; these neurones are of the pseudo-
unipolar type (see Fig. 7.2)
F – nerve fibre bundle; these consist of axons entering and
leaving the ganglion

Part C Organ systems

Gastro-intestinal system

Circulatory system

Respiratory system

Urinary system

Skeletal tissues

Nervous system

Skin

Endocrine glands

Female reproductive system

Male reproductive system

Immune system

8. Gastro-intestinal system

Introduction

The gastro-intestinal system is primarily involved in reducing food for absorption into the body. This process occurs in five main phases within defined regions of the gastro-intestinal system: (i) ingestion, (ii) fragmentation, (iii) digestion, (iv) absorption and (v) elimination of waste products. The gastro-intestinal system is essentially a muscular tract lined by a mucous membrane which exhibits regional variations in structure reflecting these progressive functions of the system from the *oral cavity* to the *anus*.

Ingestion and initial fragmentation of food occur in the oral cavity, resulting in the formation of a *bolus* of food which is then conveyed to the *oesophagus* by the action of the tongue and pharyngeal muscles during swallowing. Fragmentation and swallowing are facilitated by the secretion of *saliva* from three pairs of major *salivary glands* and numerous small accessory glands within the oral cavity. The oesophagus conducts food from the oral cavity to the *stomach* where fragmentation is completed and digestion initiated. Digestion is the process by which food is progressively broken down by enzymes into molecules which are small enough to be absorbed into the circulation; for example, ingested proteins are first broken down into polypeptides then further degraded to small peptides and amino-acids which can then be absorbed. Initial digestion, accompanied by intense muscular action of the stomach wall, reduces the stomach contents to a semi-digested liquid called *chyme*. Chyme is squirted through a muscular sphincter, the *pylorus*, into the *duodenum*, the short, first part of the *small intestine*, where it is neutralised partly by an alkaline secretion from the duodenal mucosa. Digestive enzymes from a large exocrine gland, the *pancreas*, enter the duodenum together with *bile* from the *liver* via the *common bile duct*; bile contains excretory products of liver metabolism, some of which act as emulsifying agents necessary for fat digestion. The duodenal contents pass onwards along the small intestine where the process of digestion is completed and the main absorptive phase occurs. After the duodenum, the next segment of the small intestine is called the *jejunum*; the rest of the small intestine is called the *ileum*, but there is no distinct junction between these parts of the tract.

The unabsorbed liquid residue from the small intestine passes through a valve, the *ileo-caecal valve*, into the *large intestine*. In the large intestine, water is absorbed from the liquid residue which becomes progressively more solid as it passes towards the anus. The first part of the large intestine is called the *caecum*, from which projects a blind-ended sac, the *appendix*. The major part of the large intestine is called the *colon*; the terminal portion of the large intestine, the *rectum*, is a holding chamber for faeces prior to defaecation via the *anal canal*.

Food is propelled along the gastro-intestinal tract by two main mechanisms: voluntary muscular action in the oral cavity, pharynx and upper third of the oesophagus is succeeded by involuntary waves of smooth muscle contraction called *peristalsis*. Peristalsis and the secretory activity of the entire gastro-intestinal system are modulated by the autonomic nervous system and a variety of hormones, some of which are secreted by endocrine cells located within the gastro-intestinal tract itself.

General structure of the gastro-intestinal tract

The structure of the gastro-intestinal tract conforms to a general plan which is clearly evident from the oesophagus to the anus and is illustrated in Fig. 12.20. The oral cavity and pharynx also conform to this general pattern, but this is less evident due to the extreme specialisation of these regions.

The tract is essentially a muscular tube lined by a mucous membrane. The arrangement of the major muscular component remains relatively constant throughout the tract whereas the mucosa shows marked variations in the different regions of the tract. At several points along the tract the mucosa undergoes abrupt transition from one form to another: these points are the *oesophageo-gastric junction*, the *gastro-duodenal junction*, the *ileo-caecal junction* and the *recto-anal junction*. Between these epithelial junctions the mucosa generally undergoes only a gradual transition in structure along the length of the tract.

Fig. 8.1 The gastro-intestinal system

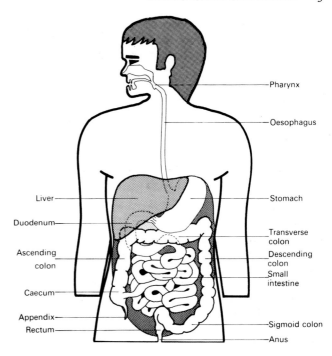

Pharynx
Oesophagus
Liver
Stomach
Duodenum
Transverse colon
Ascending colon
Descending colon
Small intestine
Caecum
Appendix
Sigmoid colon
Rectum
Anus

Fig. 8.2 General structure of the gastro-intestinal tract

The gastro-intestinal tract has four distinct functional layers: *mucosa, submucosa, muscularis* and *adventitia*.

(i) The mucosa: the mucosa is divided, histologically, into three layers: an epithelial lining, a supporting connective tissue *lamina propria* and a thin smooth muscle layer, the *muscularis mucosae*, which produces local movements and folding of the mucosa.

(ii) The submucosa: this layer of loose connective tissue supports the mucosa and contains the larger blood vessels, lymphatics and nerves.

(iii) The muscularis: this functional layer consists of smooth muscle which is subdivided usually into two histological layers: an inner circular layer and an outer longitudinal layer. The action of these smooth muscle layers, opposed at right angles to one another, is the basis of peristaltic contraction.

(iv) The adventitia: this outer layer of connective tissue conducts the major vessels and nerves. In the abdominal cavity it is continuous with the connective tissue of the mesenteries and in other sites it is continuous with the surrounding connective tissues. Where the adventitia is exposed to the abdominal cavity it is referred to as the *serosa* and is lined by a simple squamous epithelium called mesothelium.

Glands are found throughout the tract at various depths in the tract wall. In some parts of the tract, the mucosal lining is arranged into glands which have a variety of secretory functions. In some regions, glands penetrate the muscularis mucosa to lie in the submucosa. The pancreas and liver are large glands draining into the gastro-intestinal lumen but lying entirely outside the tract wall.

Lymphoid tissue is distributed throughout the tract in aggregations of variable size; these are predominantly located within the mucosal layer.

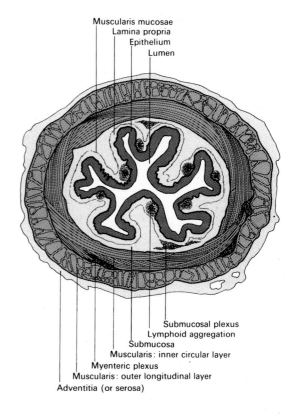

Muscularis mucosae
Lamina propria
Epithelium
Lumen

Submucosal plexus
Lymphoid aggregation
Submucosa
Muscularis: inner circular layer
Myenteric plexus
Muscularis: outer longitudinal layer
Adventitia (or serosa)

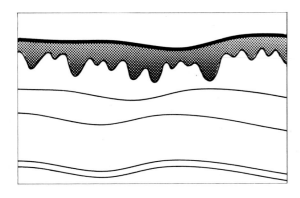

Fig. 8.3 Basic mucosal forms in the gastro-intestinal tract

There are four basic mucosal types found in the gastro-intestinal tract which can be classified according to their main function:

(a) Protective: this is found in the oral cavity, pharynx, oesophagus and anal canal; surface epithelium is stratified squamous which is keratinised in animals which have a coarse diet, e.g. rodents, herbivores.

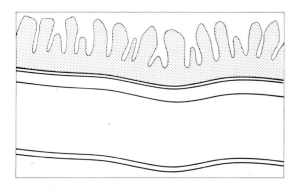

(b) Secretory: as found in the stomach; very long, closely packed, tubular glands (simple or branched depending on region of stomach).

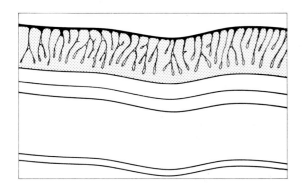

(c) Absorptive: typical of entire small intestine; mucosa folded into finger-like projections called villi (to increase surface area) with intervening short glands called crypts.

Note: in the duodenum the crypts extend through the muscularis mucosae to form submucosal mucous glands.

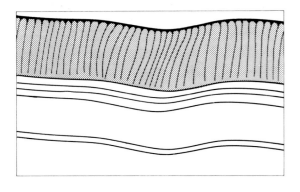

(d) Absorptive/Protective: this form lines the whole of the large intestine; mucosa arranged into closely packed straight glands consisting of cells specialised for water absorption and mucus secreting goblet cells which lubricate the passage of faeces.

Fig. 8.4 Lip and tooth

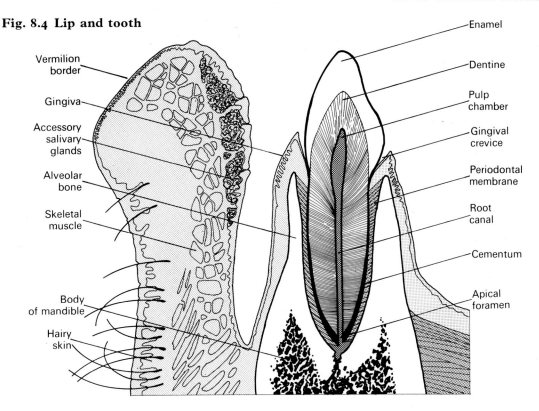

Vermilion border
Gingiva
Accessory salivary glands
Alveolar bone
Skeletal muscle
Body of mandible
Hairy skin

Enamel
Dentine
Pulp chamber
Gingival crevice
Periodontal membrane
Root canal
Cementum
Apical foramen

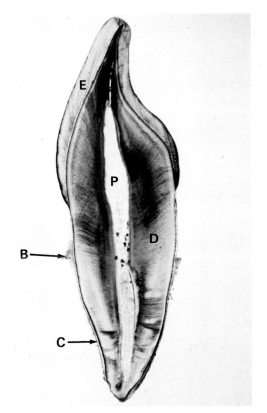

Fig. 8.5 Incisor tooth
(Undecalcified section; unstained × 5)

E – enamel; extremely hard, highly mineralised, non-cellular protective coat of tooth crown

D – dentine; forms bulk of crown and root of tooth; bone-like matrix though more highly mineralised; canalised by many minute tubules containing cytoplasmic extensions of dentine forming cells which line the pulp cavity

P – pulp cavity; in the living tooth, contains pulp consisting of highly cellular connective tissue containing many blood vessels and nerves

C – cementum; fine layer of bone-like cement substance covering tooth root; provides anchorage for dense connective tissue (periodontal membrane) which binds root to bony socket

B – bone from socket adherent after tooth extraction

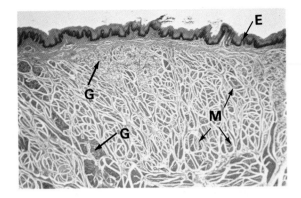

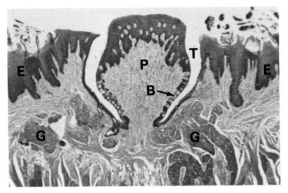

Fig. 8.6 Tongue: general structure
(H & E ×8)

E – epithelium; stratified squamous with rough keratinised surface for protection and rasping; some papillae specialised for taste and other sensation
M – interlacing bundles of skeletal muscle
G – scattered serous and mucous glands

Fig. 8.7 Circumvallate papilla on tongue
(H & E ×20)

P – circumvallate papilla; specialised projection housing taste buds (see Fig. 13.18)
T – trough surrounding papilla; harbours dissolved food for tasting
B – taste buds
E – tongue epithelium
G – serous glands draining into trough around papilla; provide solvent for tasting process

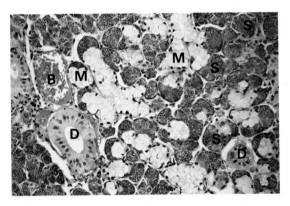

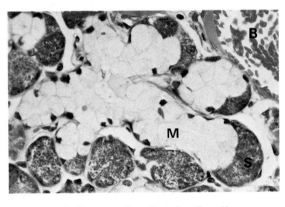

Fig. 8.8 Salivary gland (submandibular)
(H & E ×128)

S – serous gland units (strongly stained); produce amylase-rich watery secretion
M – mucous gland units (poorly stained); mucus secretion for food lubrication
D – ducts conveying saliva to mouth
B – blood vessel

Fig. 8.9 Salivary gland: mixed salivary unit
(H & E ×320)

S – serous unit
M – mucus unit
B – blood vessel

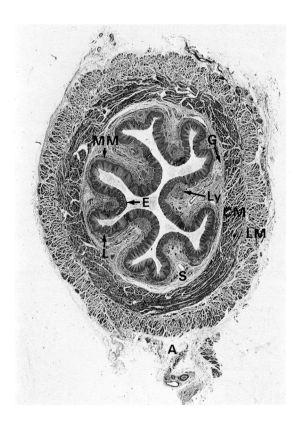

Fig. 8.10 Oesophagus
(TS: Masson's trichrome × 6)

E – epithelium; stratified squamous; folded in relaxed state allowing distention during passage of food bolus
L – lamina propria
MM – muscularis mucosae
S – submucosa
CM – circular layer of muscularis
LM – longitudinal layer of muscularis (note, upper part of oesophagus has some voluntary muscle, lower part entirely involuntary)
A – adventitia containing blood vessels
G – submucosal mucous gland (lower third only)
Ly – small lymphoid aggregation

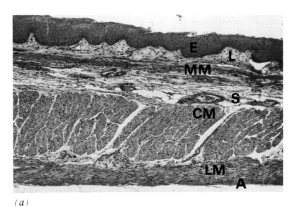

(a)

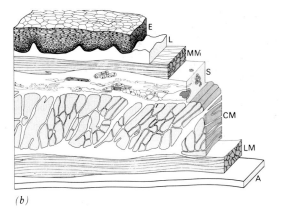

(b)

Fig. 8.11 Oesophagus
(LS: H & E × 20)

(a) LS: H & E × 20   *(b)* Explanatory diagram
E – stratified squamous epithelium
L – lamina propria
MM – muscularis mucosae
S – submucosa

CM – circular layer of muscularis
LM – longitudinal layer of muscularis
A – adventitia

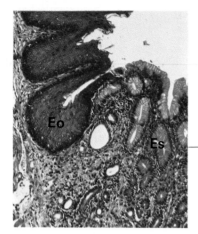

Fig. 8.13 Oesophageo-gastric junction
(H & E × 128)

Eo – oesophageal epithelium
Es – glandular epithelium of stomach

Fig. 8.12 Stomach: general structure

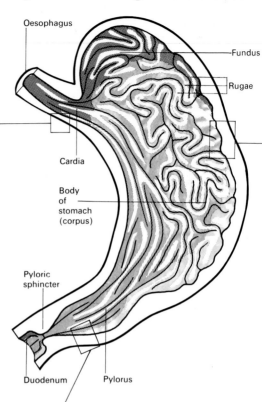

Oesophagus
Fundus
Rugae
Cardia
Body
of
stomach
(corpus)
Pyloric
sphincter
Duodenum
Pylorus

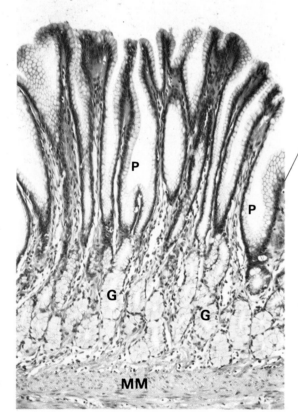

Fig. 8.14 Stomach: pyloric region
(H & E × 120)

G – branched tubular gland secreting mucus to lubricate and protect sphincter from corrosive gastric juices (note, branched glands are characteristic of the pyloric region only; rest of stomach has unbranched glands)
MM – muscularis mucosae
P – gastric pits formed by glands opening to surface

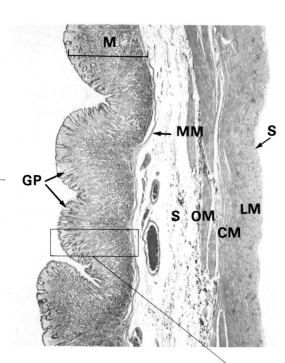

Fig. 8.15 Stomach: main body
(H & E × 12)

M – glandular mucosa containing cells secreting acid, pepsin and rennin (in children)
GP – gastric pits formed by opening of gastric glands
MM – muscularis mucosa
S – submucosa containing large arteries and veins, nerves and lymphatics
OM – oblique layer of muscularis (oblique layer is peculiar to stomach)
CM – circular layer of muscularis
LM – longitudinal layer of muscularis
S – serosa

Fig. 8.16 Gastric glands
(H & E × 120)

GP – gastric pit
M – mucus-secreting cells lining surface and gastric pits
Pl – parietal cells (characteristic 'fried egg' appearance); secrete hydrochloric acid
Pc – peptic cells (strongly stained); synthesise and secrete pepsinogen

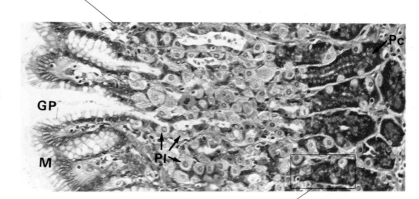

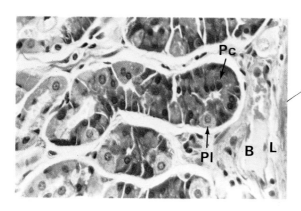

Fig. 8.17 Base of gastric gland
(H & E × 320)

Pl – parietal cells
Pc – peptic cell
B – blood vessel
L – lamina propria

Fig. 8.18 Gastro-duodenal junction

(H & E × 12)

S – stomach mucosa (glandular)
D – duodenal mucosa (villiform)
MM – muscularis mucosae
SM – submucosa
G – submucosal glands (exclusive to duodenum)
PS – pyloric sphincter; consisting of a thickening of the inner circular layer of the muscularis
CM – circular layer of muscularis
LM – longitudinal layer of muscularis
Sr – serosa

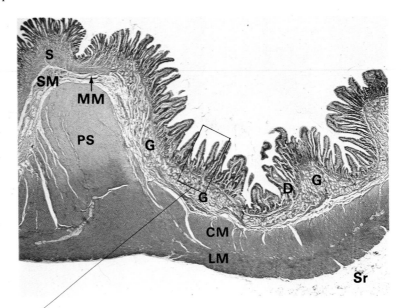

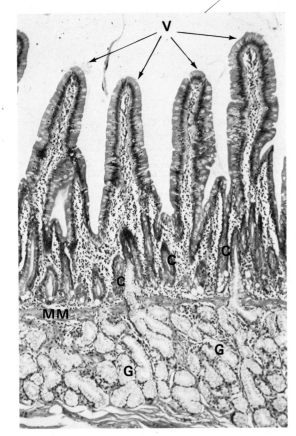

Fig. 8.19 Duodenal mucosa

(H & E × 50)

V – duodenal villi
C – duodenal crypts (crypts of Lieberkuhn); in the duodenum, some extend through muscularis mucosae to form submucosal mucous glands (Brunner's glands)
MM – muscularis mucosae
G – submucosal mucous glands (Brunner's glands)

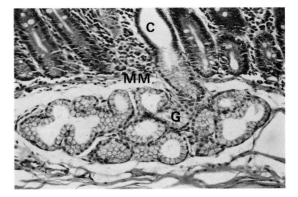

Fig. 8.20 Brunner's gland

(H & E × 128)

G – Brunner's gland; simple coiled tubular gland secreting an alkaline mucus which helps to neutralise acidic chyme from stomach
MM – muscularis mucosae
C – duodenal crypt

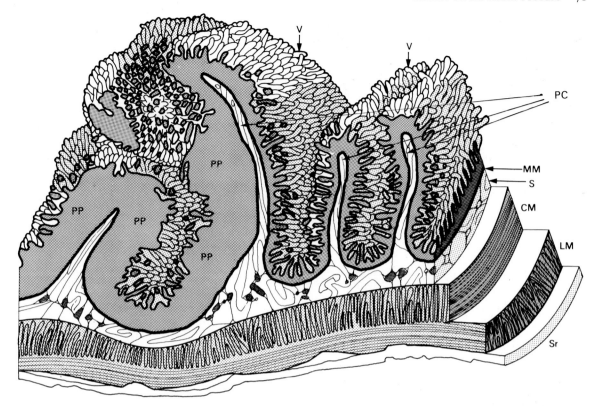

Fig. 8.21 Small intestine: general structure

The small intestine, comprising the duodenum, jejunum and ileum, is the principal site for absorption of digestion products from the gastro-intestinal tract. Digestion begins in the stomach and is completed in the small intestine in intimate association with the absorption process. Intestinal digestion occurs in two ways: *luminal digestion* and *membrane digestion*.

(i) Luminal digestion: this involves the mixing of chyme with pancreatic enzymes with subsequent molecular breakdown occurring within the intestinal lumen. Luminal digestion is greatly facilitated by adsorption of pancreatic enzymes on to the mucosal surface.

(ii) Membrane digestion: this type of digestive process involves enzymes located within the luminal plasma membranes of the cells lining the small intestine; these digestive enzymes do not occur free in the intestinal lumen.

Digestion and absorption are enhanced by the provision of an enormous surface area in the small intestine by virtue of four main features:

(a) the great length of the small intestine (four to six metres long in man);

(b) the presence of circularly arranged folds of the mucosa and submucosa called *plica circulares* or *valves of Kerckring*; the plica are particularly numerous in the jejunum;

(c) the arrangement of the mucosa into extremely numerous finger-like projections, called *villi*, and the invagination of the mucosa between the bases of the villi into crypts, called *crypts of Lieberkuhn*;

(d) the presence of extensive microvilli on the surface of each intestinal lining cell.

A prominent feature of the small intestine is the presence of lymphoid aggregations of various size within the lamina propria; the larger aggregations are known as Peyer's patches.

PC – plica circulares
V – villi
MM – muscularis mucosae
S – submucosa
CM – circular layer of smooth muscle
LM – longitudinal layer of smooth muscle
Sr – serosa
PP – Peyer's patch

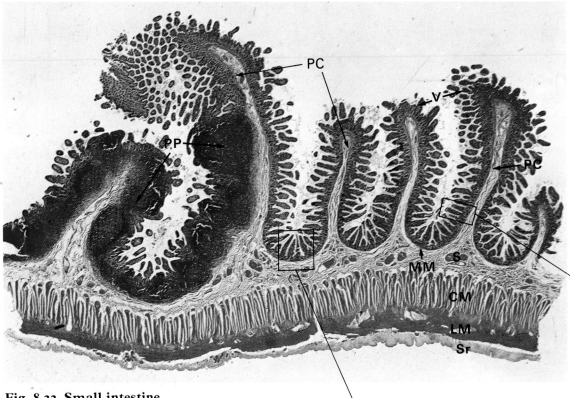

Fig. 8.22 Small intestine

(H & E × 16)

PC – plica circulares
V – villi
MM – muscularis mucosae
S – submucosa
CM – circular layer of smooth muscle
LM – longitudinal layer of smooth
muscle
Sr – serosa
PP – Peyer's patch

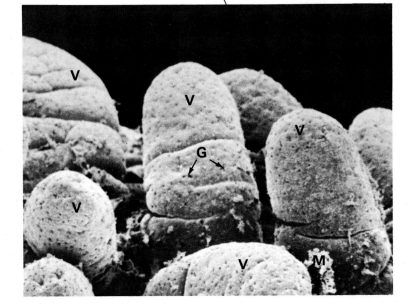

Fig. 8.23 Intestinal villi

(Scanning EM × 100)

V – villi
M – residual mucus and debris
G – goblet cell openings

Fig. 8.26 Striated border

(EM × 50000)

Mv – microvilli; projections of surface
plasma membrane which enormously
increase surface area for absorption

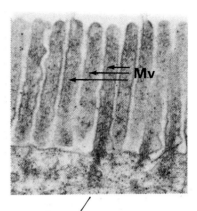

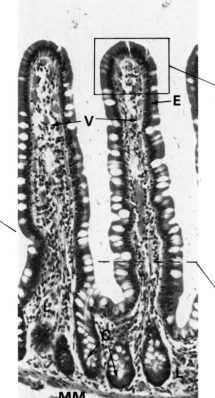

Fig. 8.24 Intestinal villi and crypts

(H & E × 120)

V – villi
E – simple tall columnar epithelium
containing absorptive cells called
enterocytes (strongly stained) and
mucus-secreting goblet cells (poorly
stained)
L – lamina propria; a core of
connective tissue forming the substance
of each villus and conducting blood
vessels and lymphatics to and from
each villus
C – crypts; epithelium of villus
produced by mitosis in the crypts then
migration along villi to be shed at the
tip
MM – muscularis mucosae

Fig. 8.25 Tip of villus

(Toluidine blue × 320)

E – enterocyte layer with goblet cells;
note cells at tip about to be shed
SB – striated border (brush border)
composed of microvilli
LP – lamina propria

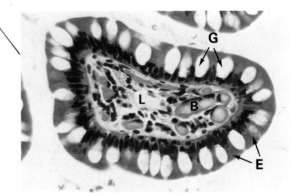

Fig. 8.27 Villus

(TS: H & E × 320)

E – enterocytes; absorptive cells
G – goblet cells
B – blood capillaries
L – lacteal; the term applied to the lymphatic vessels of
intestinal villi; lacteals convey much of the absorbed lipid
to the general circulation

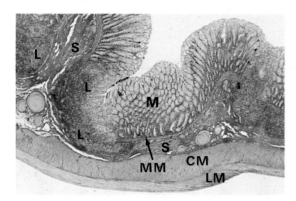

Fig. 8.28 Colon

(Alcian blue/van Gieson × 12)

M – glandular mucosa; mucus secreting cells stained green in this preparation
MM – muscularis mucosae
S – submucosa conveying large blood vessels (blood is stained yellow in this preparation)
CM – circular layer of muscularis
LM – longitudinal layer of muscularis
L – aggregation of lymphoid tissue

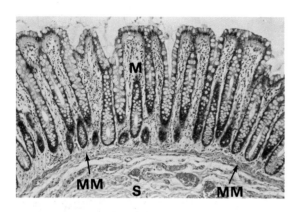

Fig. 8.29 Mucosa of the large intestine

(H & E × 50)

M – glandular mucosa; consists of simple straight tubular glands containing absorptive cells and mucus secreting (goblet) cells. Large bowel mainly involved in water absorption; mucus lubricates the passage of increasingly solid faeces
MM – muscularis mucosae
S – submucosa containing blood vessels

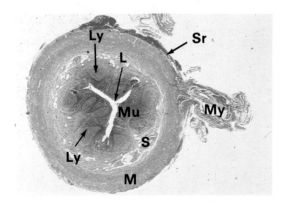

Fig. 8.30 Appendix

(TS: H & E × 5)

L – lumen; the appendix is a blind ending sac extending from the caecum
Mu – mucosa; typical of that of the rest of the large intestine
Ly – lymphoid tissue; becoming less prominent with increasing age
S – submucosa
M – muscularis (circular and longitudinal layers are difficult to distinguish in this specimen)
Sr – serosa containing blood from trauma during surgical removal
My – mesentery

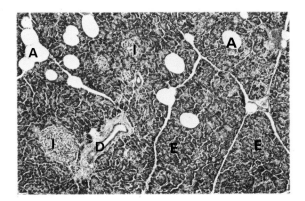

Fig. 8.31 Pancreas

(H & E × 20)

E – exocrine portion comprising bulk of the organ
(densely stained)
I – endocrine islets (Islets of Langerhans); secrete insulin
and other hormones
D – exocrine duct; conveys pancreatic secretions to
duodenum
A – adipose (fat) cells

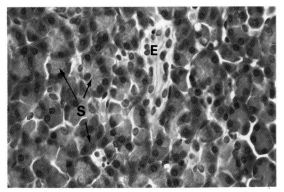

Fig. 8.32 Pancreatic exocrine tissue

(H & E × 320)

S – exocrine secretory units; composed of cells clustered
around a minute central lumen (too small to be seen in
this micrograph); the secretory cells are stained strongly
due to their large content of ribosomes which are involved
in the synthesis of pancreatic enzymes
E – small exocrine duct

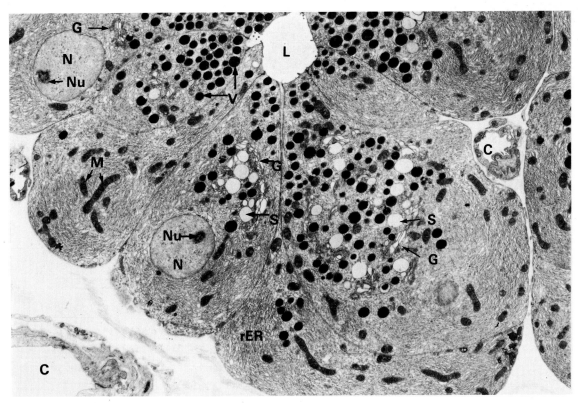

Fig. 8.33 Pancreatic secretory unit

(EM × 4270)

L – duct lumen
N – nucleus of secretory cell; note prominent nucleolus
reflecting much protein synthesis
Nu – nucleolus
rEr – rough endoplasmic reticulum; large amounts are
found in these cells, the prime function of which is the
synthesis of digestive enzymes
V – secretory vacuoles containing pancreatic enzymes
G – Golgi apparatus
S – immature secretory vesicles derived from Golgi apparatus
M – mitochondria
C – capillaries

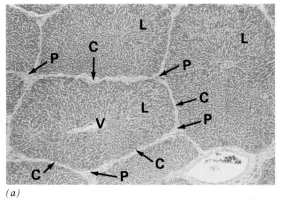

(a)

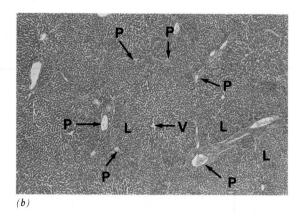

(b)

Fig. 8.34 Liver

(a) Pig liver (b) Human liver: H & E × 20

L – liver lobules; these are particularly well defined in the pig since each lobule is bounded by a distinct boundary of connective tissue, not readily seen in human liver (see Fig. 8.35)

C – connective tissue boundary to lobules

V – central vein of lobule; drains back to general circulation

P – portal tracts; convey branches of hepatic artery and hepatic portal vein passing inwards, and tributaries of the biliary system passing outwards; in the human liver the portal tracts define the boundaries of the lobules

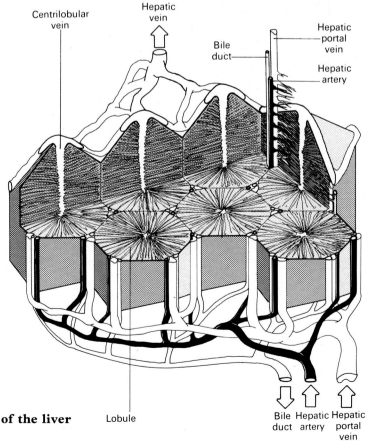

Fig. 8.35 Lobular architecture of the liver showing blood and bile flow

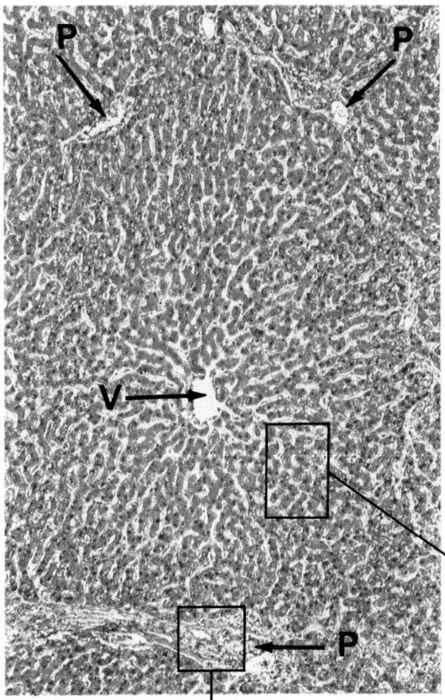

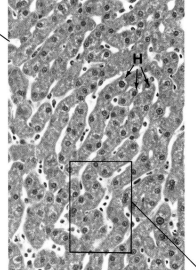

Fig. 8.36 Liver lobule
(Human: H & E × 50)

P – portal tract
V – central vein

Fig. 8.37 Liver parenchyma
(H & E × 198)
H – hepatocytes; arranged in branching plates one cell thick and separated by broad capillaries known as sinusoids

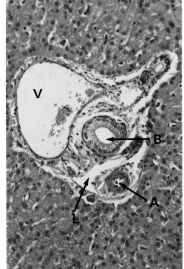

Fig. 8.39 Portal tract
(H & E × 128)

V – branch of hepatic portal vein; conducts absorbed food products from the gastro-intestinal tract
A – branch of hepatic artery; supplies oxygenated blood to the liver from the aorta
B – small bile duct; lined by simple, tall cuboidal epithelium; collects bile produced by hepatocytes and conveys this to the duodenum via the large common bile duct
L – lymphatic vessel

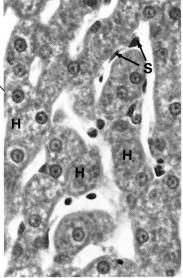

Fig. 8.38 Hepatocytes
(H & E × 480)

H – hepatocytes; note the large nuclei with prominent nucleoli reflecting the great metabolic activity of the liver; the cytoplasm is strongly stained due to its high content of mitochondria and ribosomes
S – sinusoid lining cells; some of these cells are involved in phagocytosis of particulate matter from blood, e.g. aged or damaged red blood cells

9. Circulatory system

Introduction

The circulatory system mediates the continuous movement of all body fluids; its principal functions are the transport of oxygen and nutrients to the tissues and transport of carbon dioxide and other metabolic waste products from the tissues. The circulatory system is also involved in temperature regulation and the distribution of molecules such as hormones, and cells such as those of the immune system. The circulatory system has two functional components: the blood vascular system and the lymph vascular system. The *blood vascular system* constitutes a circuit of vessels through which a flow of blood is maintained by continuous pumping of the heart. The *arterial system* provides a distribution network to the *capillaries* which are the main sites of interchange between the tissues and blood. The *venous system* returns blood from the capillaries to the heart. In contrast, the *lymph vascular system* is merely a passive drainage system for returning excess extravascular fluid called *lymph* to the blood vascular system. The lymph vascular system has no intrinsic pumping mechanism.

The whole circulatory system has a common basic structure:

(i) an inner lining comprising a single layer of extremely flattened epithelial cells called *endothelium* supported by a basement membrane and connective tissue;

(ii) an intermediate smooth muscle layer containing a variable amount of elastin;

(iii) an outer connective tissue layer which becomes continuous with the surrounding tissue.

The muscular layer exhibits the greatest variation throughout the system; for example, it is more or less absent in capillaries but comprises almost the whole mass of the heart. Blood flow is predominantly influenced by variations in activity of the muscular layer. In the heart, the cardiac muscle provides a pumping mechanism. In blood vessels the muscular layer regulates vessel diameter and thus permits blood flow to different organs to be varied in accordance with functional needs.

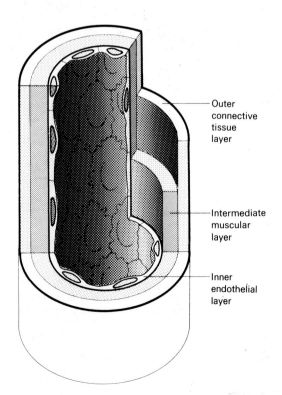

Outer connective tissue layer

Intermediate muscular layer

Inner endothelial layer

Fig. 9.1 General structure of vascular system

The basic differences between arteries, veins and capillaries are summarised as follows:

(a) Arteries: (small diameter arteries are known as arterioles): muscular layer predominates; larger arteries, e.g. aorta, also contain much elastin.

(b) Veins: (small veins are known as venules): muscular layer is thin but easily discernible, outer connective tissue forms the thickest layer. Valves consist of flaps of endothelium with a very delicate connective tissue core.

(c) Capillaries: (large diameter capillaries are often referred to as sinusoids): endothelial cells are the major component; only a few smooth muscle cells; outer connective tissue layer completely merges with surrounding tissues.

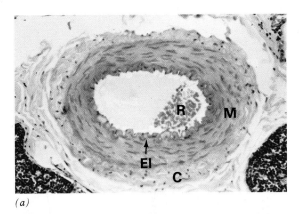

(a)

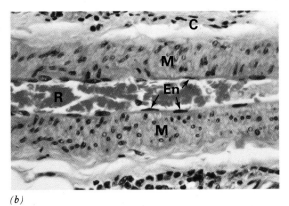

(b)

Fig. 9.2 Arterial system

(a) Muscular artery, T.S: (H & E ×128)
(b) Muscular artery, L.S: (H & E ×320)
(c) Elastic artery, e.g. aorta: (Elastic van Gieson ×80)

En – endothelium
M – smooth muscle layer
C – outer connective tissue layer
El – layer of elastin concentrated at inner aspect of muscular layer; elastin (stained black in *(c)*) also scattered throughout muscular layer and outer connective tissue layer
R – red blood cells

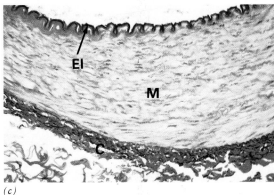

(c)

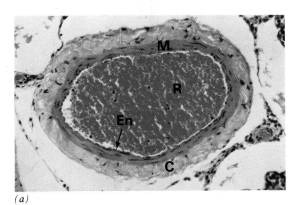

(a)

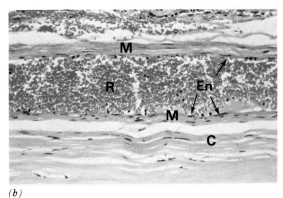

(b)

Fig. 9.3 Venous system

(a) Vein, T.S: (H & E ×128)
(b) Vein, L.S: (H & E ×128)
(c) Vein with valve: (Masson's trichrome ×128)

En – endothelium
M – smooth muscle layer
C – outer connective tissue layer
V – valve flaps
R – red blood cells

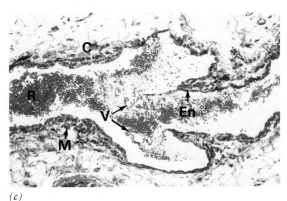

(c)

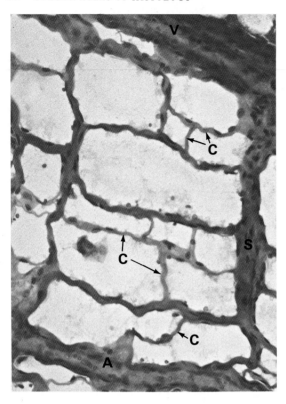

Fig. 9.4 Capillary bed
(Mesenteric spread preparation; H & E × 120)

A – arteriole
V – venule
S – arteriovenous shunt (bypasses capillary network)
C – capillaries

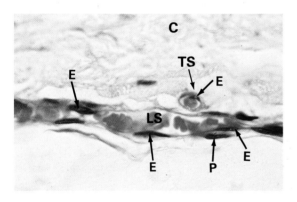

Fig. 9.5 Capillaries
(H & E × 800)

LS – capillary in longitudinal section
TS – capillary in transverse section
E – endothelial cell nuclei
C – connective tissue
P – pericyte; probably contractile

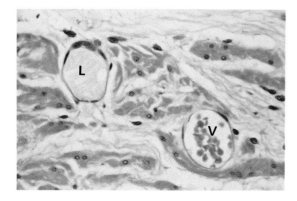

Fig. 9.6 Venule and small lymphatic vessel
(H & E × 320)

L – lymphatic vessel
V – venule

Note: venules contain erythrocytes whereas lymphatics contain amorphous protein material from tissue fluid (and often lymphocytes, though not in this micrograph).

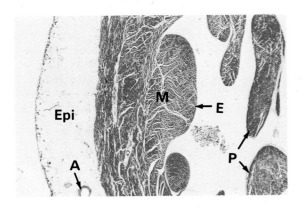

Fig. 9.7 Heart: wall of ventricle
(Masson's trichrome × 20)

Epi – epicardium (visceral pericardium)
M – myocardium
A – branch of coronary artery
E – endocardium
P – papillary muscles (act as 'guy ropes' for interventricular valves)

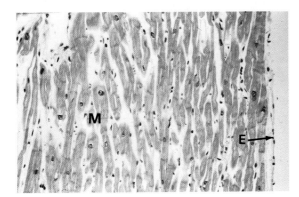

Fig. 9.8 Myocardium and endocardium
(H & E × 128)

M – myocardium
E – endocardium; lined by endothelium

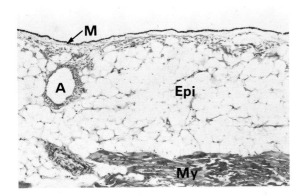

Fig. 9.9 Epicardium
(H & E × 128)

My – myocardium
Epi – epicardium; mainly composed of adipose tissue
A – branches of coronary artery
M – mesothelial lining of pericardial cavity; simple squamous epithelium

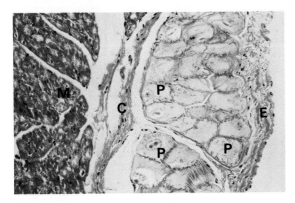

Fig. 9.10 Purkinje fibres
(Masson's trichrome × 128)

M – myocardium
P – Purkinje fibres; highly specialised cardiac muscle fibres which conduct contraction impulse from atrio-ventricular node throughout ventricle
C – connective tissue
E – endocardium

10. Respiratory system

Introduction

Respiration is a term used to describe two different but interrelated processes: cellular respiration and mechanical respiration. Cellular respiration is the process in which cells derive energy by degradation of organic molecules (see Chapter 1). Mechanical respiration is the process by which oxygen required for cellular respiration is absorbed from the atmosphere into the blood vascular system and the process by which carbon dioxide is excreted into the atmosphere. Mechanical respiration occurs within the respiratory system.

The respiratory system has two functional components: a conducting system for transport of inspired and expired gases between the atmosphere and the circulatory system, and an interface for passive exchange of gases between the atmosphere and blood. The conducting system begins essentially as a single tube which divides repeatedly to form airways of ever decreasing diameter. The terminal branches of the conducting system open into blind-ended sacs called *alveoli*, which are the sites of gaseous exchange. The alveoli, which constitute the bulk of the lung tissue, are thin-walled structures enveloped by a rich network of capillaries. This arrangement provides a vast interface of minimal thickness for gaseous exchange between the atmosphere and blood. The continuous process of gaseous diffusion requires appropriate gaseous pressure gradients to be maintained across the alveolar wall. This is achieved by rapid and continuous perfusion of the pulmonary capillaries by venous blood and regular replacement of alveolar gases in breathing.

The respiratory system is divided anatomically into two parts, the *upper* and *lower respiratory tracts*, which are separated by the *pharynx*.

The lower respiratory tract begins at the *larynx* then continues into the thorax as the *trachea* before dividing into numerous orders of smaller airways to reach the alveoli. The vocal cords of the larynx protect the lower respiratory tract against the entry of foreign bodies, in addition to performing a vital function in speech. The vocal cords are the only part of the lower respiratory tract which is not lined by respiratory epithelium; they are lined by stratified squamous epithelium which is better adapted to withstand frictional stress. The trachea first divides into left and right *main bronchi* which supply the lungs. Each main bronchus further divides into various smaller bronchi which then ramify into numerous orders of progressively smaller airways called *bronchioles*, the smallest of which mark the end of the purely conducting portion of the tract. The terminal bronchioles branch further into a series of transitional airways, which become increasingly involved in gaseous exchange. These passages finally open into the alveoli.

Each type of airway has its own characteristic structural feature but there is a gradual, rather than abrupt, transition from one type of airway to the next along the whole length of the tract. In general terms, the airways are pliable tubes lined by respiratory mucosa and containing variable amounts of muscle and/or cartilage. The principal structural features of the lower respiratory tract are as follows:

(a) The respiratory epithelium undergoes progressive transition from a tall, pseudostratified columnar, ciliated form in the larynx and trachea to a simple, cuboidal, non-ciliated form in the smallest airways. Goblet cells are numerous in the trachea but decrease in number and are absent in the smaller bronchioles.

(b) The epithelium is supported by fibro-elastic connective tissue which contains lymphoid aggregations of variable size and density; these form part of the immune defence system (see Chapter 18).

(c) A layer of smooth muscle lies deep to the mucosa (except in the trachea) and becomes increasingly prominent as the airway diameter decreases; it reaches its greatest prominence in the smallest bronchioles. Smooth muscle tone controls the diameter of the conducting passages and thus controls resistance to air flow within the respiratory tree. Smooth muscle tone is modulated by the autonomic nervous system, adrenal medullary hormones and local factors.

(d) Submucosal connective tissue underlies the smooth muscle layer and contains serous and mucous glands which become progressively less numerous in the narrower airways and are not present beyond the bronchi.

(e) Cartilage provides a supporting skeleton for the larynx, trachea and bronchi and prevents the collapse of these airways during ventilation. This layer lies outside the submucosa and diminishes in prominence as the calibre of the airway decreases.

(f) The outermost layer of cartilage or smooth muscle is surrounded by fibro-elastic connective tissue which merges with surrounding tissues.

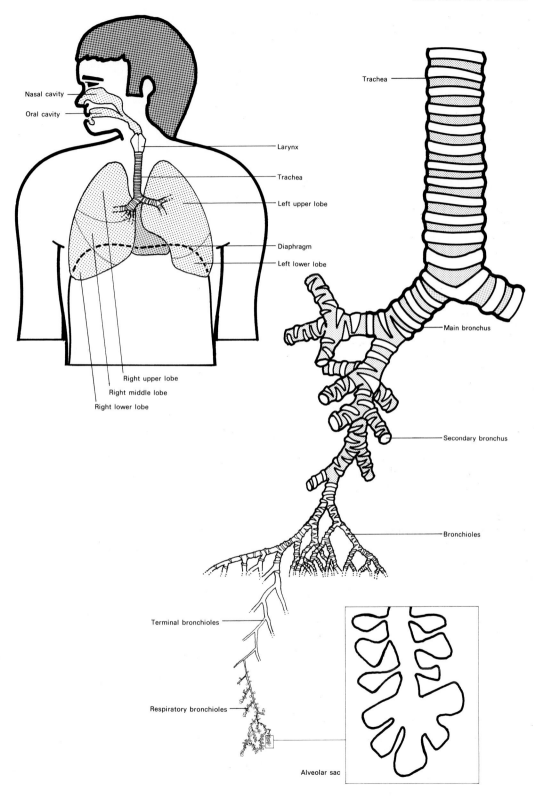

Nasal cavity

Oral cavity

Larynx

Trachea

Left upper lobe

Diaphragm

Left lower lobe

Right upper lobe

Right middle lobe

Right lower lobe

Trachea

Main bronchus

Secondary bronchus

Bronchioles

Terminal bronchioles

Respiratory bronchioles

Alveolar sac

Fig. 10.1 Structure of respiratory system

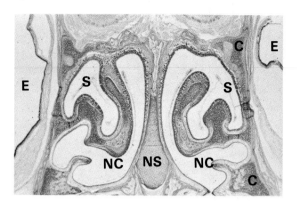

Fig. 10.2 Nasal cavity

(Kitten: coronal section; H & E/Alcian blue ×8)

NS – nasal septum; mainly composed of cartilage (stained blue)
NC – nasal cavity; lined by nasal mucosa
S – sinus; lined by nasal mucosa
E – eye cavity
C – cartilage of developing facial skeleton

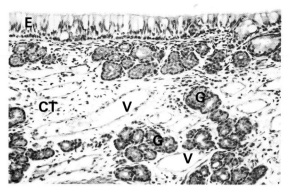

Fig. 10.3 Nasal mucosa

(H & E ×128)

E – pseudostratified columnar ciliated epithelium with goblet cells; mucus traps inhaled dust particles
CT – loose supporting connective tissue
V – venules; blood warms inspired air
G – serous glands; provide watery fluid to humidify inspired air

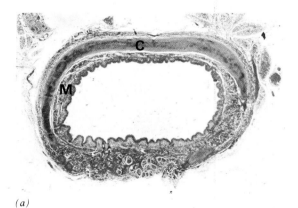

(a)

Fig. 10.4 Trachea

(a) T.S: H & E/Alcian blue ×6
(b) Tracheal mucosa: H & E ×198

C – tracheal cartilage ring (not seen in (b))
M – tracheal mucosa
E – pseudostratified columnar ciliated epithelium with goblet cells
BM – basement membrane
CT – supporting fibro-elastic connective tissue
G – mixed serous and mucous glands
P – outer layer of cartilagenous ring (perichondrium)

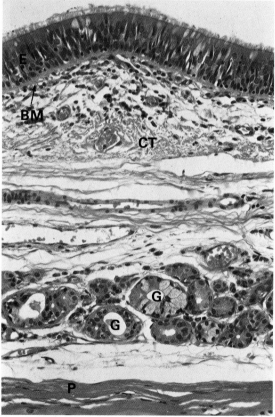

(b)

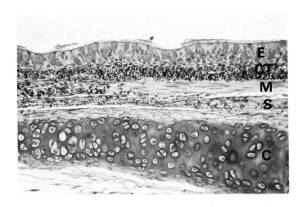

Fig. 10.5 Main bronchus
(Elastic van Gieson/Alcian blue ×80)

E – pseudostratified columnar ciliated epithelium
CT – supporting fibro-elastic connective tissue
M – smooth muscle layer
S – submucosal connective tissue
C – cartilage

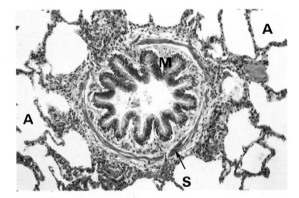

Fig. 10.6 Small bronchus
(Elastic van Gieson ×90)

E – respiratory epithelium
M – smooth muscle layer
C – cartilage; little cartilagenous support remains at this level
G – glands; very few glands at this level
L – lymphoid aggregation; part of immune system
A – alveoli

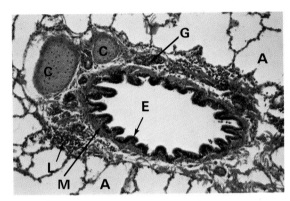

Fig. 10.7 Bronchiole
(H & E ×80)

M – bronchiolar mucosa
S – smooth muscle layer
A – alveoli

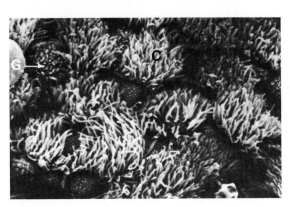

Fig. 10.8 Respiratory epithelium
(Scanning EM ×2000)

C – cilia
G – goblet cell openings

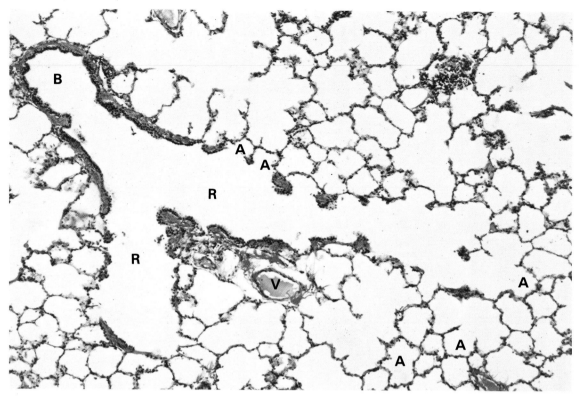

Fig. 10.9 Terminal portion of the respiratory tree

(Elastic van Gieson × 40)

B – smallest, purely conducting, bronchiole
R – first part of gaseous exchange system and terminal portion of conducting system (respiratory bronchiole)
A – alveoli
V – vein

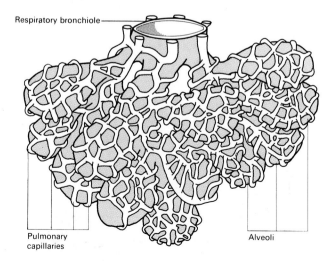

Fig. 10.10 Lung capillary network

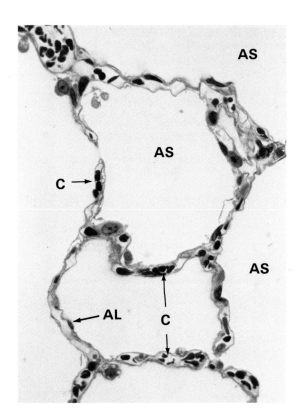

Fig. 10.11 Alveoli
(Toluidine blue × 480)

AS – alveolar air space
AL – alveolar lining cell; simple squamous epithelium
C – alveolar capillary

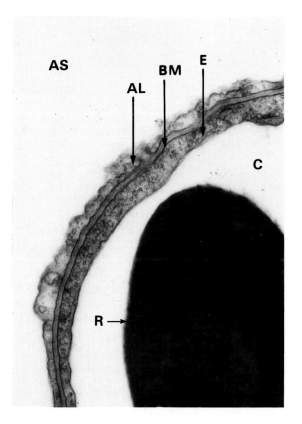

Fig. 10.12 Gaseous diffusion barrier
(EM × 30 000)

AS – alveolar air space
AL – cytoplasm of alveolar lining cell
BM – basement membrane shared by alveolar lining cell and capillary lining cell
C – capillary lumen
R – red blood cell
E – cytoplasm of capillary lining cell

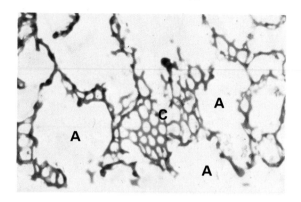

Fig. 10.13 Lung capillary network
(Dye-perfused preparation × 420)

C – 'basket' of capillaries surrounding an alveolus
A – alveolar space

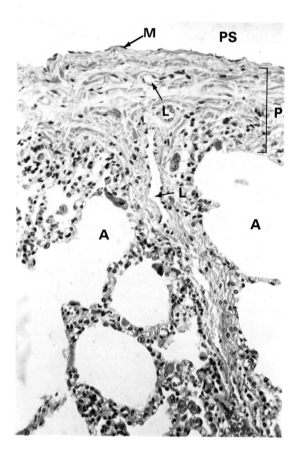

Fig. 10.14 Pleural surface of lung
(H & E × 198)

P – pleura; composed of connective tissue containing many blood and lymphatic vessels
M – mesothelium; simple squamous epithelium lining the pleural cavity and outer surface of the lung
PS – pleural space; in life this is only a potential space
A – alveoli
L – lymphatic vessels

11. Urinary system

Introduction

The urinary system is the principal organ system responsible for water and electrolyte homeostasis. The maintenance of homeostasis requires that any input into a system is balanced by an equivalent output; the urinary system provides the mechanism by which excess water and electrolytes are eliminated from the body. A second major function of the urinary system is the excretion of many toxic metabolic waste products, particularly the nitrogenous compounds urea and creatinine; this excretory function is intimately related to water and electrolyte elimination which provides an appropriate fluid vehicle. The end product of these processes is *urine*. Since all body fluids are maintained in dynamic equilibrium with one another via the circulatory system, any adjustment in the composition of the blood is reflected in complementary changes in the other fluid compartments of the body. Thus regulation of the osmotic potential of blood plasma ensures the osmotic regulation of all other body fluids. This process, primarily performed by the urinary system, is called *osmoregulation*.

The functional units of the urinary system are the *nephrons*, of which there are approximately one million in each human kidney. Nephrons perform the functions of osmoregulation and excretion by the following processes:

(i) filtration of most relatively small molecules from blood plasma to form a filtrate;

(ii) selective reabsorption of most of the water and other molecules from the filtrate, leaving behind excess and waste materials to be excreted;

(iii) secretion of some excretory products directly from blood into the filtrate.

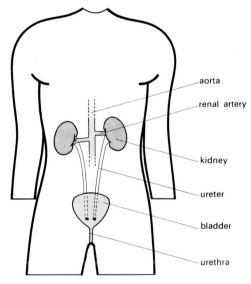

Fig. 11.1 The urinary system

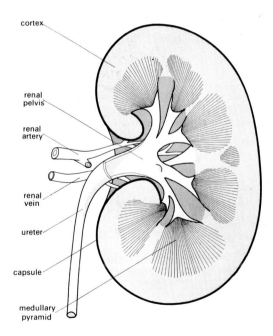

Fig. 11.2 Kidney

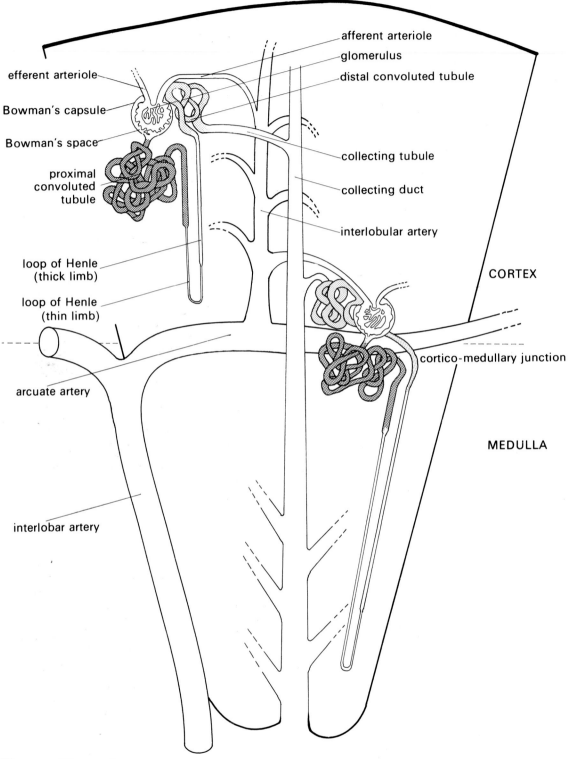

Fig. 11.3 The nephron

Fig. 11.3 The nephron *(illustration opposite)*

The nephron, the functional unit of the kidney, consists of two major components, the *renal corpuscle* and the *renal tubule*.

(i) Renal corpuscle: the renal corpuscle is that part of the nephron responsible for the filtration of plasma and is a combination of two structures, *Bowman's capsule* and the *glomerulus*.

(a) Bowman's capsule consists of a single layer of flattened cells resting on a basement membrane; it forms the distended, blind end of an epithelial tubule, the renal tubule.

(b) The glomerulus is a tightly coiled network of anastomosing capillaries which invaginates Bowman's capsule. Within the capsule, the glomerulus is invested by a layer of epithelial cells, called *podocytes*, which constitutes the *visceral layer of Bowman's capsule*; the visceral layer is reflected around the vascular stalk of the glomerulus to become continuous with the *parietal layer*, the Bowman's capsule proper (see Fig. 11.4). The space between the visceral and parietal layers is known as *Bowman's space* and is continuous with the lumen of the renal tubule; the parietal epithelium of Bowman's capsule is continuous with the epithelium lining the renal tubule.

In the renal corpuscle, elements of plasma are filtered from the glomerular capillaries into Bowman's space, and the *glomerular filtrate* then passes into the renal tubule. Thus the filtration barrier between the capillary lumen and Bowman's space consists of the capillary endothelium, the podocyte layer and a common basement membrane, the *glomerular basement membrane*, separating these two cellular layers.

The *afferent arteriole* supplies the glomerulus, and the *efferent arteriole* drains the glomerulus.

(ii) Renal tubule: the renal tubule extends from Bowman's capsule to its junction with a *collecting duct*. The renal tubule is up to 55mm long in man and is lined by a single layer of epithelial cells. The primary function of the renal tubule is the selective reabsorption of water, inorganic ions and other molecules from the glomerular filtrate. In addition, some inorganic ions are secreted directly from blood into the lumen of the tubule. In man, glomerular filtrate is produced at a steady rate of approximately 120 cm^3 per minute; of this, approximately 119 cm^3 per minute are reabsorbed in the renal tubules. The highly convoluted renal tubule has four distinct histo-physiological zones, each of which has a different role in tubular function.

(a) *The proximal convoluted tubule (PCT):* this is the longest, most convoluted section of the tubule; PCTs make up the bulk of the renal cortex. Approximately seventy-five per cent of all the ions and water of the glomerular filtrate are reabsorbed from the PCT.

(b) *The loop of Henle:* this arises from the PCT as a straight, thin-walled limb (*the thin limb*) which descends from the cortex into the medulla; here it loops closely back on itself to ascend as a straight, thicker-walled limb (*the thick limb*) into the renal cortex. The limbs of the loop of Henle are closely associated with parallel, wide capillary loops which arise from glomerular efferent arterioles, descend into the medulla then loop back on themselves to drain into veins at the junction of the medulla and cortex. The main function of the loops of Henle is to generate a high osmotic potential in the extracellular fluid of the renal medulla; the mechanism by which this is achieved is known as the *counter-current multiplier system*.

(c) *The distal convoluted tubule (DCT):* this is shorter and less convoluted than the PCT. Sodium ions are actively reabsorbed from the DCT by a process which is controlled by the adreno-cortical hormone *aldosterone*.

(d) *The collecting tubule:* this is the terminal portion of the DCT and conducts urine to the *collecting ducts* which merge to form large ducts in the renal medulla. The collecting tubules and ducts are not normally permeable to water; however, in the presence of antidiuretic hormone (ADH), secreted by the posterior pituitary, the collecting tubules and ducts become permeable to water which is then drawn out by the high osmotic potential of the medullary extracellular fluid; reabsorbed water is then returned to the general circulation.

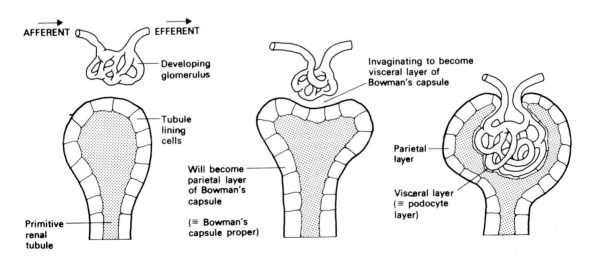

Fig. 11.4 Development of the renal corpuscle

(Highly schematic)

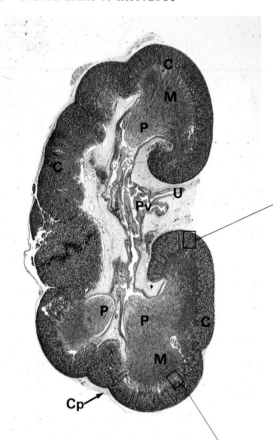

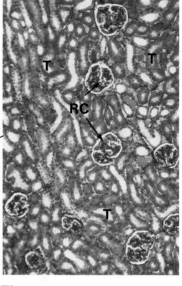

Fig. 11.6 Renal cortex
(Azan ×80)

RC – renal corpuscles
T – various renal tubules, mainly proximal and distal convoluted tubules

Fig. 11.5 Kidney
(Newborn child: H & E ×3)

C – renal cortex; site of most renal corpuscles
M – medulla; mainly composed of loops of Henle, collecting tubules and ducts and blood vessels
P – renal papilla; large collecting ducts pass through the papilla to drain into the renal pelvis
Pv – renal pelvis; collecting space for urine; drains into ureter
U – ureter
Cp – tough connective tissue capsule

Fig. 11.7 Cortico-medullary junction

CD – collecting ducts; from the cortex the collecting ducts converge to form bundles before entering the medulla
RC – small corpuscles in extensions of the cortex lying between bundles of collecting ducts
V – blood vessels

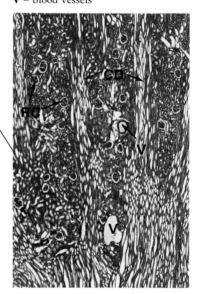

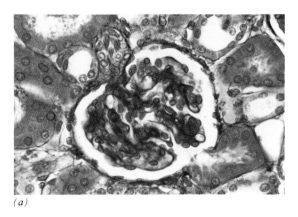

(a)

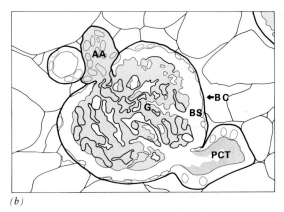

(b)

Fig. 11.8 Renal corpuscle

(a) Azan × 320 (b) explanatory diagram

AA – afferent arteriole
BC – Bowman's capsule
BS – Bowman's space
PCT – proximal convoluted tubule
G – glomerulus

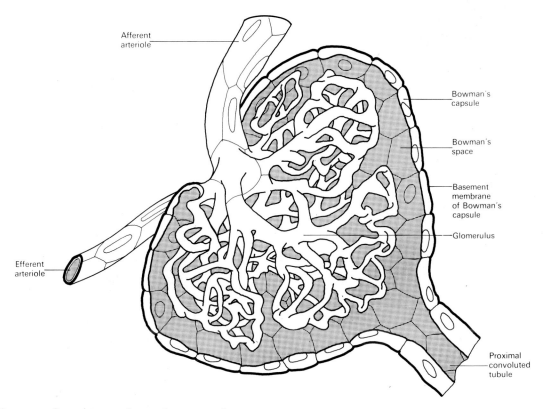

Afferent arteriole

Bowman's capsule

Bowman's space

Basement membrane of Bowman's capsule

Glomerulus

Efferent arteriole

Proximal convoluted tubule

Fig. 11.9 Structure of renal corpuscle

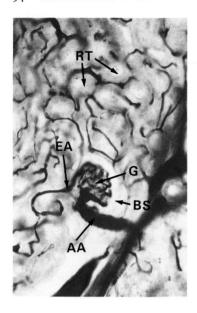

Fig. 11.10 Blood supply of glomerulus

(Carmine-gelatine perfused × 128)

AA – afferent arteriole
EA – efferent arteriole
G – glomerulus
BS – Bowman's space
RT – renal tubules; note that these are also surrounded by capillaries which return reabsorbed filtrate to the general circulation

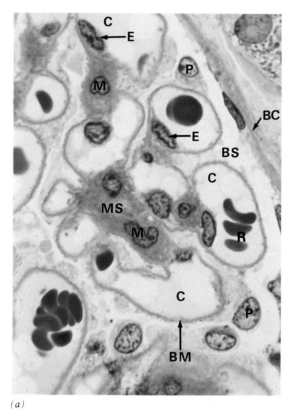

(a)   *(b)*

Fig. 11.11 Glomerulus

(a) Toluidine blue × 1200 (b) explanatory diagram

C – glomerular capillary lumen
E – capillary endothelial cell nuclei
R – red blood cells
P – podocyte nucleus
BM – glomerular basement membrane, i.e. shared by podocytes and capillary endothelial cells
BC – Bowman's capsule
BS – Bowman's space
M – mesangial cells; provide support for glomerular capillaries
MS – mesangial substance; produced by mesangial cells

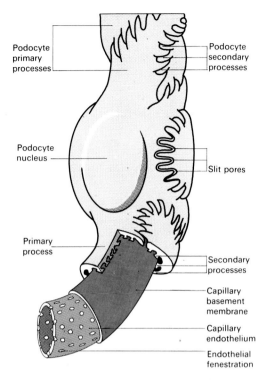

Fig. 11.12 Components of the glomerular filter

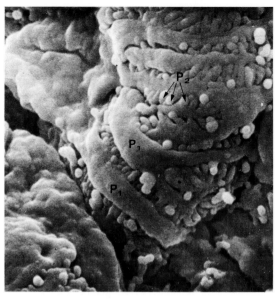

Fig. 11.13 Podocytes
(Scanning EM × 4500)

P₁ – podocyte primary foot processes
P₂ – podocyte secondary foot processes

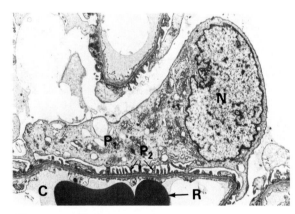

Fig. 11.14 Podocyte
(EM × 4275)

N – podocyte nucleus
P₁ – primary foot processes
P₂ – secondary foot processes
C – capillary lumen
R – red blood cell

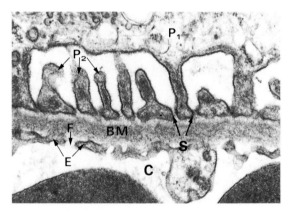

Fig. 11.15 Slit pores and glomerular basement membrane

P₁ – podocyte primary foot processes
P₂ – podocyte secondary foot processes
S – slit pores
BM – basement membrane
E – capillary endothelial cytoplasm
F – capillary endothelial fenestration
C – capillary lumen

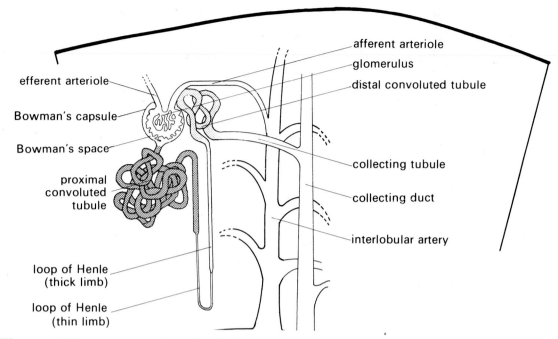

afferent arteriole

glomerulus

distal convoluted tubule

efferent arteriole

Bowman's capsule

Bowman's space

proximal
convoluted
tubule

collecting tubule

collecting duct

interlobular artery

loop of Henle
(thick limb)

loop of Henle
(thin limb)

Fig. 11.16 Components of renal tubule

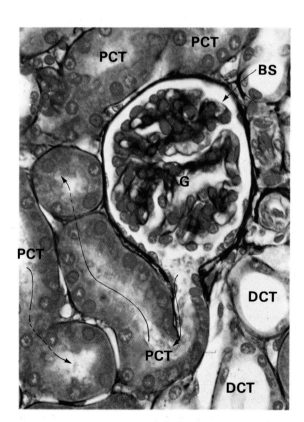

Fig. 11.17 Proximal convoluted tubule

(Azan × 48)

PCT – proximal convoluted tubules; note brush border
BS – Bowman's space
G – glomerulus
DCT – distal convoluted tubules

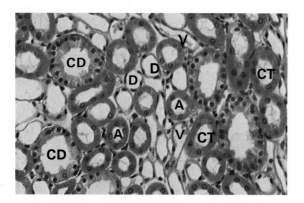

Fig. 11.18 Loop of Henle

(H & E × 198)

D – descending limbs of loop of Henle
A – ascending limbs of loop of Henle
CT – collecting tubules
CD – collecting ducts
V – blood vessels; loop into medulla and make up counter-current multiplier system

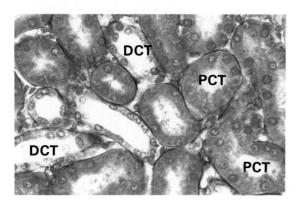

Fig. 11.19 Distal convoluted tubule

(Azan × 320)

DCT – distal convoluted tubule; no brush border and wider lumen than PCT
PCT – proximal convoluted tubule

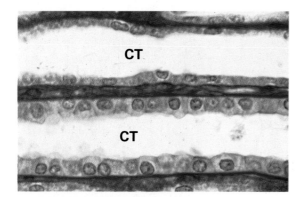

Fig. 11.20 Collecting tubules

(Azan × 500)

CT – collecting tubules; upper tubule is more proximal hence lower cuboidal epithelium

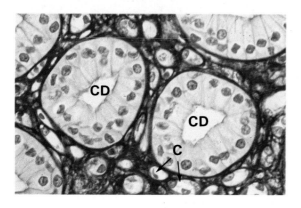

Fig. 11.21 Collecting ducts

(Azan × 320)

CD – collecting ducts
C – capillaries

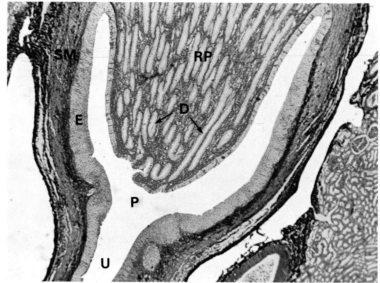

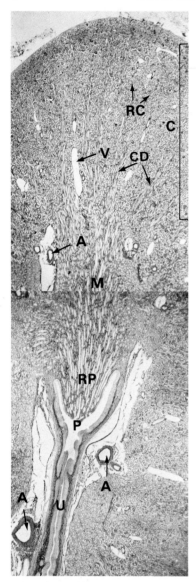

Fig. 11.23 Renal papilla

(Azan ×30)

RP – renal papilla; contains large collecting ducts **D** which drain into pelvis
P – renal pelvis
U – ureter
E – transitional epithelium
SM – smooth muscle layer; note this is continuous with the smooth muscle of the ureter

Fig. 11.22 Segment of a kidney

(Monkey: Jones' methenamine silver ×8)

C – renal cortex
RC – renal corpuscles
CD – collecting ducts
V – veins
A – arteries
RP – renal papilla
M – renal medulla
P – renal pelvis
U – ureter

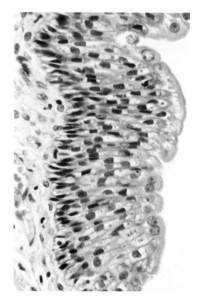

Fig. 11.24 Transitional epithelium

(H & E ×320)

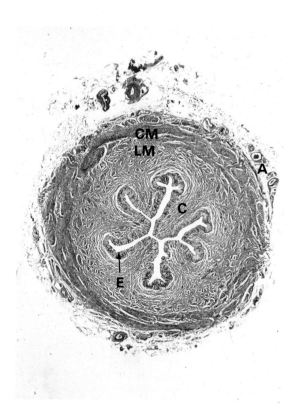

Fig. 11.25 Ureter
(Masson's trichrome × 12)

E – transitional epithelium
C – supporting connective tissue (collagen stained blue-green)
LM – inner longitudinal layer of smooth muscle
CM – outer circular layer of smooth muscle
A – outer adventitial layer of connective tissue

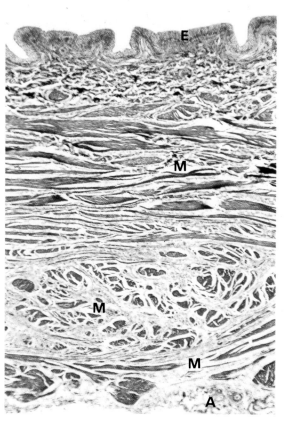

Fig. 11.26 Urinary bladder
(Masson's trichrome × 12)

E – transitional epithelium
M – smooth muscle; arranged loosely into three layers: inner longitudinal, intermediate circular and outer longitudinal
A – outer adventitial layer of connective tissue

12. Skeletal tissues

Introduction

The skeletal system is composed of a variety of specialised forms of connective tissue. Bone provides a rigid protective and supporting framework for most of the soft tissues of the body, whereas cartilage provides semi-rigid support in limited sites such as the respiratory tree and external ear. Joints are composite structures which unite the bones of the skeleton and, depending on their structure, permit varying degrees of movement of the skeleton. Ligaments are flexible bands which contribute to the stability of joints. Tendons provide strong, flexible connections between muscles and their points of insertion into bones.

The functional differences between the various tissues of the skeletal system relate principally to the different nature and proportion of the ground substance and fibrous elements of the extracellular matrix. The cells of all the skeletal tissues, like the cells of connective tissues in general, have close structural and functional relationships and a common origin from primitive mesodermal cells.

Cartilage

Cartilage is a semi-rigid form of connective tissue, the characteristics of which mainly stem from the nature and predominance of ground substance in the extracellular matrix. Glycoproteins, containing a high proportion of sulphated polysaccharide units, make up the ground substance and account for the solid, yet flexible, property of cartilage.

Within the ground substance are embedded varying proportions of collagen and elastic fibres giving rise to three main types of cartilage: *hyaline cartilage, fibro-cartilage* and *elastic cartilage.*

Cartilage formation commences with the differentiation of stellate-shaped, primitive mesodermal cells to form rounded cartilage precursor cells called *chondroblasts.* Subsequent mitotic divisions give rise to aggregations of closely packed chondroblasts which grow and begin synthesis of ground substance and fibrous extracellular material. Secretion of extracellular material traps each chondroblast in a space or *lacuna* within the cartilagenous matrix thereby separating the chondroblasts from one another. Each chondroblast then undergoes one or two further mitotic divisions to form a small group of mature cells separated by a small amount of extracellular material. Mature cartilage cells, known as *chondrocytes,* maintain the integrity of the cartilage matrix. This differentiation and maturation sequence is most advanced in the centre of a mass of growing cartilage. Towards the periphery of the cartilage, chondroblasts, at progressively earlier stages of differentiation, merge with the surrounding loose connective tissue. On completion of growth, the cartilage mass consists of chondrocytes embedded in a large amount of extracellular matrix. At the periphery of mature cartilage is a zone of condensed connective tissue called *perichondrium*, containing chondroblasts with cartilage-forming potential. Growth of cartilage occurs by *interstitial growth* from within and *appositional growth* at the periphery.

In mature mammals, cartilage has a limited distribution, whereas in immature mammals cartilage occurs more extensively since it forms a template for most of the developing bony skeleton.

The three different forms of cartilage differ in the following respects:

(i) Hyaline cartilage: this is the most common type and is found in the nasal septum, tracheal rings, most articular surfaces and sternal ends of the ribs. It is also the form of cartilage in the templates which precede the formation of many of the bones of the skeleton. Mature hyaline cartilage is characterised by small aggregations of chondrocytes embedded in an amorphous matrix of ground substance reinforced by collagen fibres.

(ii) Elastic cartilage: this occurs in the external ear and external auditory canal, the epiglottis, parts of the laryngeal cartilages and the walls of the Eustacean tubes. The histological structure of elastic cartilage is similar to that of hyaline cartilage; its elasticity however, derives from the presence of numerous bundles of branching elastic fibres in the cartilage matrix.

(iii) Fibrocartilage: this has features intermediate between cartilage and dense fibrous connective tissue; it is found in the intervertebral discs, some articular cartilages, the pubic symphysis, and in association with dense connective tissue in joint capsules, ligaments and the connections of some tendons to bone. Fibrocartilage consists of alternating layers of hyaline cartilage matrix containing chondrocytes and thick layers of dense collagen fibres oriented in the direction of the functional stresses.

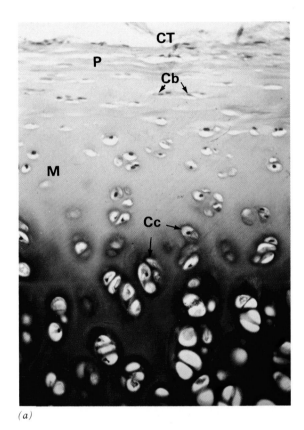

(a)

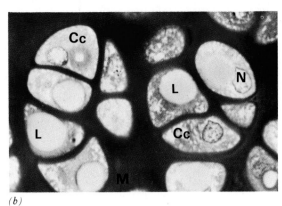

(b)

Fig. 12.1 Hyaline cartilage

(a) H & E × 78 (b) Toluidine blue × 800

P – perichondrium
Cb – chondroblasts
M – cartilage matrix
CT – surrounding connective tissue
Cc – chondrocytes in lacunae
N – chondrocyte nuclei
L – cytoplasmic lipid droplets in chondrocytes

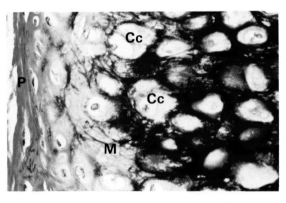

Fig. 12.2 Elastic cartilage

(Elastic van Gieson × 128)

P – perichondrium
Cc – chondrocytes
M – cartilage matrix; elastin stains black with this technique

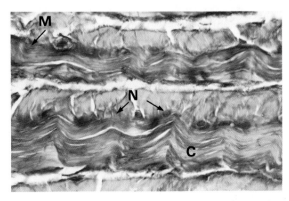

Fig. 12.3 Fibrocartilage

(H & E/Alcian blue × 320)

N – chondrocyte nuclei
C – collagen (stained pink)
M – cartilage matrix (stained blue)

Bone

Bone is a specialised form of connective tissue in which the extracellular components are mineralised, thus conferring the property of marked rigidity and strength whilst retaining some degree of elasticity. In addition to its supporting and protective function, bone constitutes a variable store of calcium and other inorganic ions, and actively participates in the maintenance of calcium homeostasis in the body as a whole. The structure of individual bones provides for the maximum resistance to mechanical stresses whilst maintaining the least bony mass. To accommodate changing mechanical stresses and the demands of calcium homeostasis, all bones in the body are in a dynamic state of growth and resorption throughout life. Like other connective tissues, bone is composed of cells and an organic extracellular matrix containing glycoprotein ground substance and collagen fibres. Inorganic salts, predominantly *calcium hydroxyapatite* crystals, form the mineral component of bone matrix.

The cells found in bone are of three types: *osteoblasts, osteocytes* and *osteoclasts*. These three cell types are derived from, and may revert to less differentiated cells called *osteoprogenitor cells*. Osteoblasts are immature forms of bone cells and are responsible for the synthesis and secretion of the organic component of the extracellular matrix of bone, a substance known as *osteoid*; osteoid then rapidly undergoes mineralisation to form bone. Osteoblasts become trapped within bone as osteocytes and are then responsible for maintenance of the bone matrix. Osteoclasts are multinucleate cells formed by the fusion of numerous osteoprogenitor cells, and are actively involved in resorptive processes associated with continuous remodelling of bone.

Ground substance constitutes only a small proportion of the organic extracellular matrix of bone and contains glycoproteins similar to those found in cartilage. The proportion of sulphated glycoproteins is much less than in cartilage. The fibrous component of the extracellular material is mainly collagen.

Bone exists in two main forms: *woven bone* and *lamellar bone*. Woven bone is an immature form and is characterised by a random (woven) organisation of its fibrous elements. During bone development, woven bone is the first form of bone to be produced; it is then remodelled to form lamellar bone, the form which constitutes most of the mature skeleton. Lamellar bone is composed of successive layers each of which has a highly organised infrastructure. Lamellar bone may be formed as a solid mass, when it is described as *compact bone*, or may be formed as a spongy mass, described as *cancellous bone*.

Bone development and growth

The fetal development of bone occurs in two ways, both of which involve replacement of connective tissues by bone. The resulting woven bone is then extensively remodelled by resorption and appositional growth to form the mature adult skeleton which is made up of lamellar bone. Thereafter, resorption and deposition of bone occur at a much reduced rate to accommodate changing functional stresses and to effect calcium homeostasis. The bones of the vault of the skull, the maxilla and most of the mandible are formed by the deposition of bone within primitive mesodermal tissue; this process of direct replacement of mesenchyme by bone is known as *intramembranous ossification* and the bones so formed are called *membrane bones*. In contrast, the long bones, vertebrae, pelvis and bones of the base of the skull are preceded by the formation of a continuously growing cartilage model which is progressively replaced by bone; this process is called *endochondral ossification* (see Fig. 12.11) and the bones so formed are called *cartilage bones*. Bone development is controlled by growth hormone, thyroid hormone and the sex hormones.

Fig. 12.4 Long bone

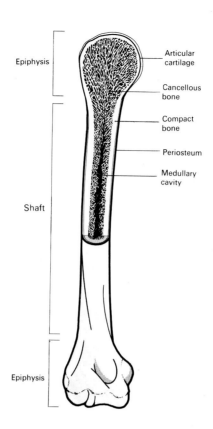

Epiphysis

Articular
cartilage

Cancellous
bone

Compact
bone

Periosteum

Medullary
cavity

Shaft

Epiphysis

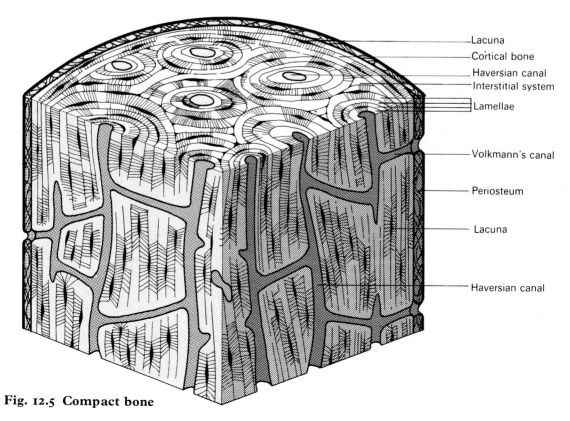

Lacuna

Cortical bone

Haversian canal

Interstitial system

Lamellae

Volkmann's canal

Periosteum

Lacuna

Haversian canal

Fig. 12.5 Compact bone

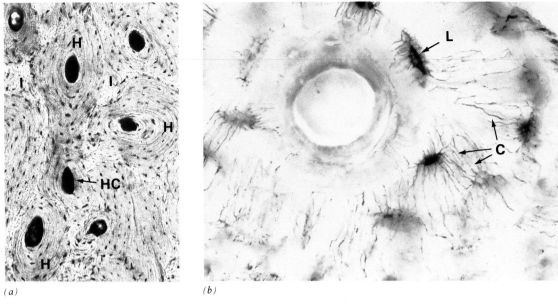

(a)   (b)

Fig. 12.6 Compact bone

(Ground sections, unstained: (a) ×80 (b) ×480)

H – Haversian system
HC – Haversian canal
I – interstitial system
L – lacuna; osteocytes destroyed in preparation
C – canaliculi; minute canals in bone which interconnect
the lacunae and Haversian canals

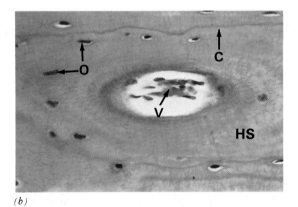

(b)

Fig. 12.7 Compact bone

(Decalcified section: H & E (a) ×198 (b) ×320)

HS – Haversian system
HC – Haversian canal
I – interstitial system
C – cement lines; represent rest periods between
deposition of successive lamellae of compact bone
CB – cortical bone
O – osteocyte
V – blood vessels in Haversian canal

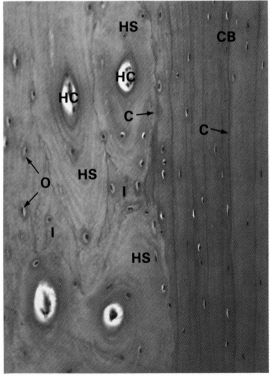

(a)

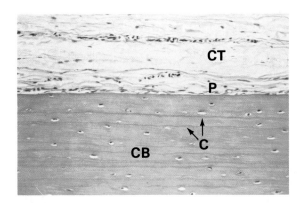

Fig. 12.8 Cortical bone and mature periosteum

(H & E ×128)

CB – cortical bone
C – cement lines
P – periosteum
CT – surrounding connective tissue

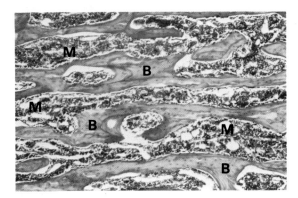

Fig. 12.9 Cancellous bone

(Skull: H & E ×50)

B – bony trabeculae; composed of irregular lamellae of bone with lacunae containing osteocytes
M – bone marrow; site of blood cell formation

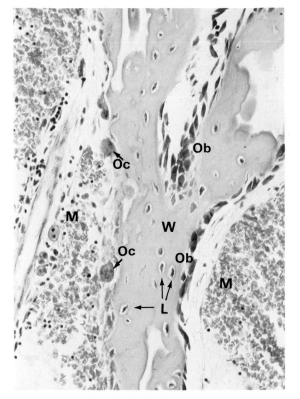

Fig. 12.10 Bone remodelling

(H & E ×480)

W – woven bone matrix
L – lacunae containing osteocytes
Ob – osteoblasts; laying down new bone
Oc – osteoclasts; multinucleate cells involved in resorption of bone
M – bone marrow

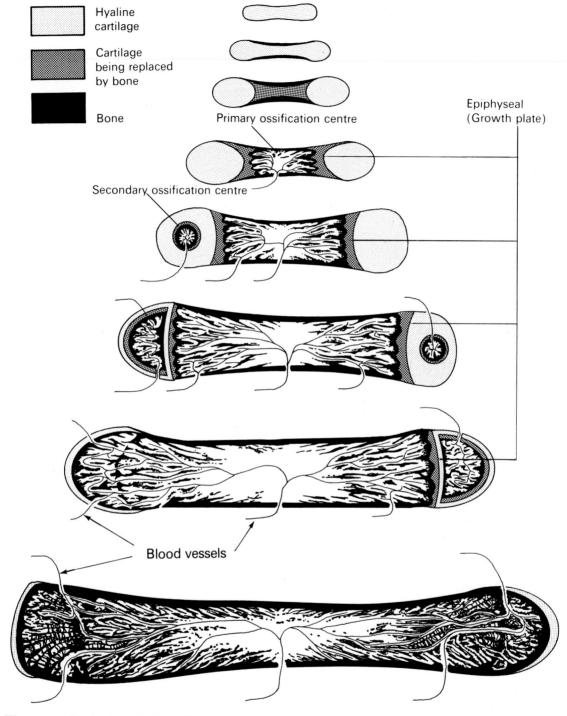

Fig. 12.11 Endochondral ossification

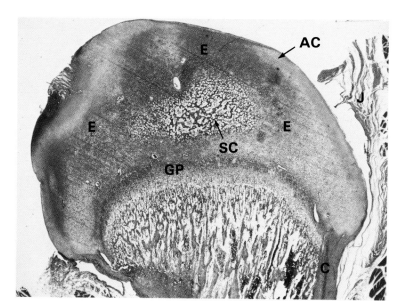

Fig. 12.12 Endochrondral ossification: epiphysis

(H & E/Alcian blue × 12)

E – epiphysis (hyaline cartilage)
GP – growth plate
SC – secondary ossification centre in epiphysis
AC – articular cartilage (hyaline)
J – joint capsule
C – cortical bone of shaft

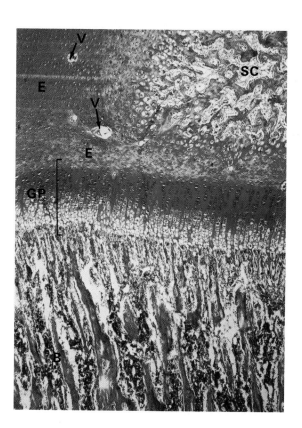

Fig. 12.13 Endochondral ossification: epiphyseal growth plate

(H & E/Alcian blue × 30)

GP – growth plate
E – epiphyseal hyaline cartilage
SC – secondary centre of ossification
V – blood vessels supplying secondary ossification centre
B – newly forming bone of shaft

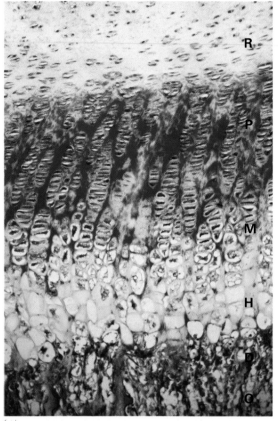

(a)

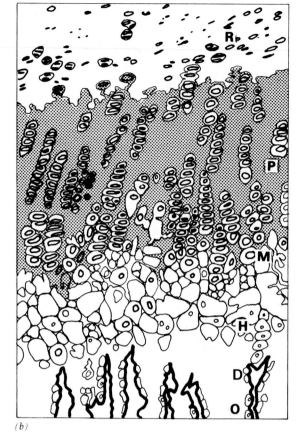

(b)

Fig. 12.14 Endochondral ossification: epiphyseal growth plate

(a) H & E/Alcian blue × 120   (b) Explanatory diagram

R – zone of reserve cartilage
P – zone of proliferation of chondrocytes
M – zone of maturation of chondrocytes
H – zone of chondrocyte hypertrophy and matrix calcification

D – zone of chondrocyte degeneration
O – zone of bone formation on template formed by degenerate cartilage

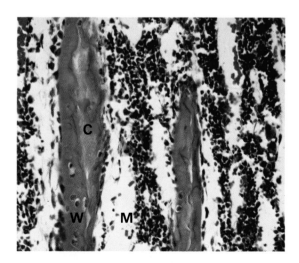

Fig. 12.15 Endochondral ossification: new bone formation

(H & E/Alcian blue × 198)

C – calcified cartilage matrix (stained blue); forms framework for new bone deposition; cartilage matrix will be later completely resorbed and replaced by bone.
W – newly formed woven bone (stained pink)
M – bone marrow

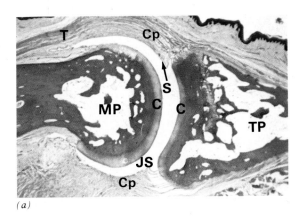

(a)

Fig. 12.16 Synovial joint

(a) Finger joint of monkey: H & E × 12
(b) Articular cartilage: H & E × 128

C – articular cartilage
TP – terminal phalangeal bone
MP – middle phalangeal bone
Cp – joint capsule
JS – joint space
T – tendon to terminal phalanx
S – synovial membrane; lines joint capsule and produces lubricating synovial fluid

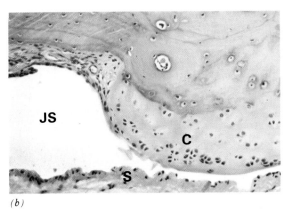

(b)

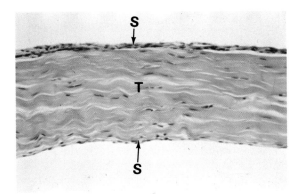

Fig. 12.17 Tendon

(H & E × 128)

T – tendon; extremely dense regular connective tissue
S – tendon sheath

13. Nervous system

Central nervous tissues

The central nervous system consists of the brain and spinal cord, each of which can be divided grossly into areas of so-called *grey matter* and *white matter*; grey matter contains almost all the neurone cell bodies and their associated fibres, whereas white matter consists merely of tracts of nerve fibres. Central nervous tissue consists of a vast number of neurones and their processes embedded in a mass of support cells, collectively known as *neuroglia*; there is little intercellular matrix.

The outer surface of the brain and spinal cord is covered by three specialised connective tissue layers, the dura mater, arachnoid mater and pia mater respectively, collectively known as the *meninges*. Although each functional zone of the CNS has its own peculiar histological appearance, the basic organisation of grey and white matter remains consistent throughout; only the principles of organisation are discussed in this section.

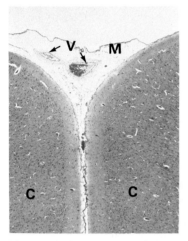

Fig. 13.1 Cerebral cortex

(H & E ×20)

C – cerebral cortex; consists of many layers of neurones of different functional types
M – meninges
V – meningeal blood vessel

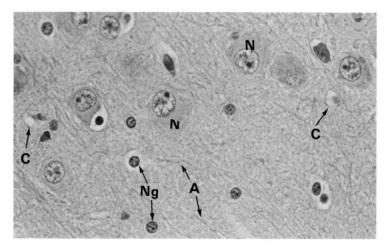

Fig. 13.2 Cerebral cortex

(H & E ×480)

N – neurone cell bodies
Ng – neuroglia of various different types; these provide support to the neurone cell bodies and axons
A – axons
C – cerebral capillaries

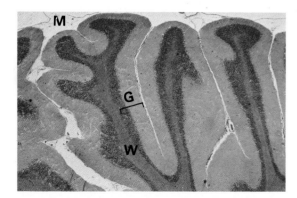

Fig. 13.3 Cerebellum

(H & E ×8)

G – cerebellar grey matter; made up of two distinct layers of neurone cell bodies
W – cerebellar white matter; made up of axons passing to and from cortex
M – meninges of cerebellum

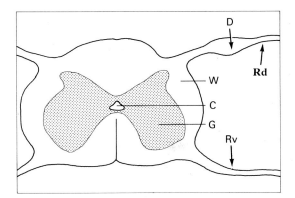

Fig. 13.4 Spinal cord

W – white matter; contains mainly axons
G – grey matter; contains nerve cell bodies
D – dorsal root ganglion; contains cell bodies of general sensory neurones
Rd – dorsal nerve root; conveys afferent sensory fibres
Rv – ventral nerve root; conveys efferent motor fibres
C – central canal

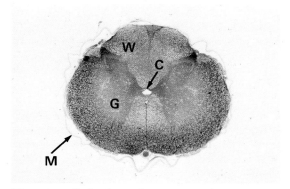

Fig. 13.5 Spinal cord

(Gold method × 8)

W – white matter
G – grey matter
C – central canal
M – meninges of spinal cord

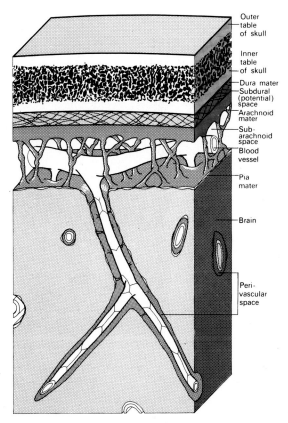

Fig. 13.6 Meninges

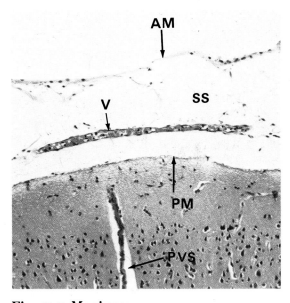

Fig. 13.7 Meninges

(H & E × 198)

AM – arachnoid mater; note the skull and dura mater have been removed
SS – subarachnoid space
PM – pia mater
V – subarachnoid blood vessel
PVS – perivascular space surrounding penetrating vessel

Peripheral nervous tissues

Peripheral nerves are anatomical structures which may contain any combination of afferent or efferent nerve fibres of either the somatic or autonomic nervous systems. The cell bodies of fibres coursing in peripheral nerves are either located in the CNS or in ganglia in peripheral sites.

Each peripheral nerve is composed of one or more bundles of nerve fibres; within the bundles, each individual nerve fibre, with its investing Schwann cell, is surrounded by a delicate packing of loose connective tissue which contains a few fibroblasts and blood capillaries. Each nerve bundle is surrounded by a condensed layer of collagenous connective tissue. In peripheral nerves consisting of more than one bundle, a further layer of loose connective tissue binds the bundles together and is condensed peripherally to form a cylindrical sheath. The larger blood vessels supplying the nerve are found within the outer connective tissue layer. The fibres within a peripheral nerve derive considerable mechanical strength from these three layers of connective tissue.

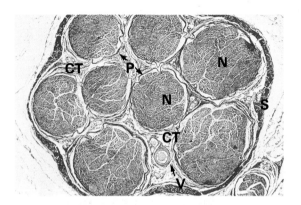

Fig. 13.8 Large peripheral nerve
(T.S: van Gieson × 20)

N – nerve bundle containing many thousands of nerve fibres
CT – connective tissue separating the nerve bundles
V – blood vessel in supporting connective tissue
S – tough connective tissue sheath surrounding the nerve
P – connective tissue sheath investing individual nerve fibre

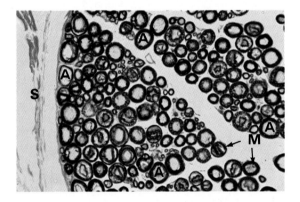

Fig. 13.9 Fibres in peripheral nerve
(T.S: Osmium fixation: van Gieson × 800)

A – axons; note marked variation in diameter of different fibres subserving different sensory and motor functions
M – myelin sheaths (stain black after osmium fixation); also very variable in thickness; some axons are not myelinated
S – connective tissue sheath of fibre bundle

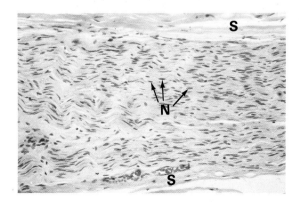

Fig. 13.10 Peripheral nerve
(L.S: H & E × 128)

N – nuclei of Schwann cells (plus occasional fibroblast nuclei from delicate supporting connective tissue); note wavy course of fibres which permits stretching
S – connective tissue sheath

Organs of sensory reception

Sensory receptors are nerve endings or specialised cells which convert (transduce) stimuli from the external or internal environments into afferent nerve impulses; the impulses pass into the CNS where they initiate appropriate voluntary or involuntary responses.

No classification system for sensory receptors has yet been devised which adequately incorporates either functional or morphological features. A widely used functional classification divides sensory receptors into three groups: *exteroceptors*, *proprioceptors* and *interoceptors*. Exteroceptors are those which respond to stimuli from outside the body, and include separate receptors for touch, light pressure, deep pressure, cutaneous pain, temperature, smell, taste, sight and hearing. Proprioceptors are located within the skeletal system and provide conscious and unconscious information about orientation, skeletal position, tension and movement; such receptors include the vestibular apparatus of the ear, tendon organs and neuromuscular spindles. Interoceptors respond to stimuli from the viscera and include the chemoreceptors of blood, vascular baroreceptors, the receptors for the state of distension of hollow viscera such as the gastro-intestinal tract and urinary bladder, and receptors for such nebulous senses as visceral pain, hunger, thirst, well-being and malaise.

The nature of the receptors involved in some of these sensory modalities is poorly understood; however, sensory receptors may be classified morphologically into two groups: *simple* and *compound*. Simple receptors are merely free, branched or unbranched nerve endings such as those responsible for cutaneous pain and temperature. Simple receptors are rarely visible with the light microscope unless special staining methods are employed. Compound receptors involve organisation of non-neural tissues to complement the function of neural receptors. The degree of organisation may range from mere encapsulation to highly sophisticated arrangements such as in the eye.

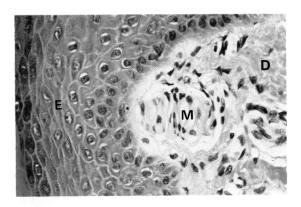

Fig. 13.11 Meissner's corpuscle

(H & E ×320)

M – Meissner's corpuscle; encapsulated sensory organ in dermis of skin; responsible for reception of light touch sensation
D – dermis
E – epidermis

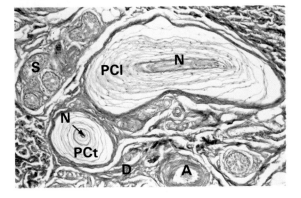

Fig. 13.12 Pacinian corpuscles

(Masson's trichrome ×80)

PCl – Pacinian corpuscle; LS
PCt – Pacinian corpuscle; TS
N – central nerve fibre; senses vibration, pressure or coarse touch which is amplified by concentric layers of connective tissue and interstitial fluid
D – dermis
S – sweat glands
A – dermal arteriole

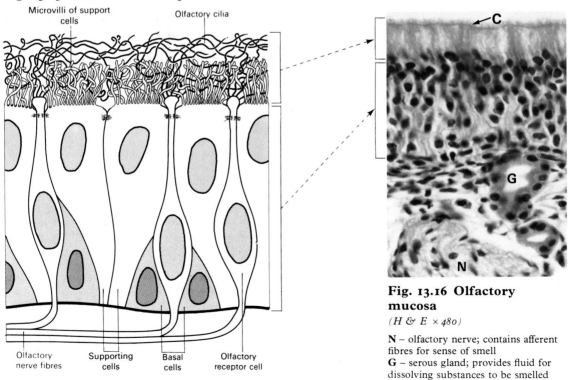

Motor nerve to
spindle muscle
fibres

Muscle
fibres

Spindle muscle
fibres

Capsule

Sensory nerves
from spindle

Motor nerve to
skeletal muscle
fibres

Fig. 13.13 Neuromuscular spindle

Fig. 13.14 Neuromuscular spindle

(LS: H & E × 320)

C – capsule of spindle
F – muscle fibres of spindle
M – skeletal muscle fibres

Microvilli of support cells

Olfactory cilia

Olfactory
nerve fibres

Supporting
cells

Basal
cells

Olfactory
receptor cell

Fig. 13.15 Olfactory receptors

Fig. 13.16 Olfactory mucosa

(H & E × 480)

N – olfactory nerve; contains afferent
fibres for sense of smell
G – serous gland; provides fluid for
dissolving substances to be smelled
C – cilia

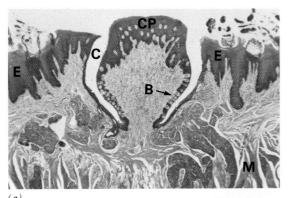

(a)

Fig. 13.17 Taste receptors

(H & E (a) ×20 (b) ×128 (c) ×1200)

B – taste buds
CP – circumvallate papilla of tongue
C – cleft surrounding circumvallate papilla
E – tongue epithelium
M – tongue muscle
TP – taste pore

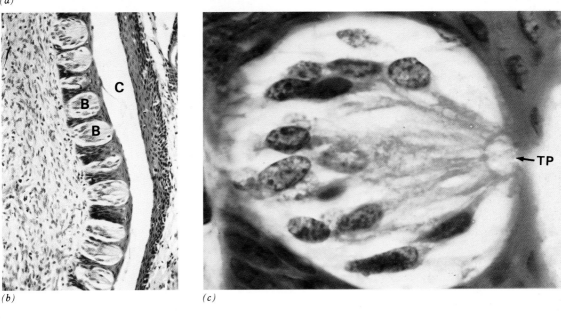

(b)

(c)

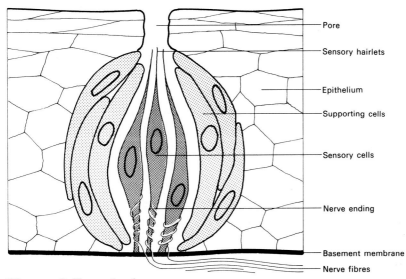

Pore

Sensory hairlets

Epithelium

Supporting cells

Sensory cells

Nerve ending

Basement membrane

Nerve fibres

Fig. 13.18 Taste bud structure

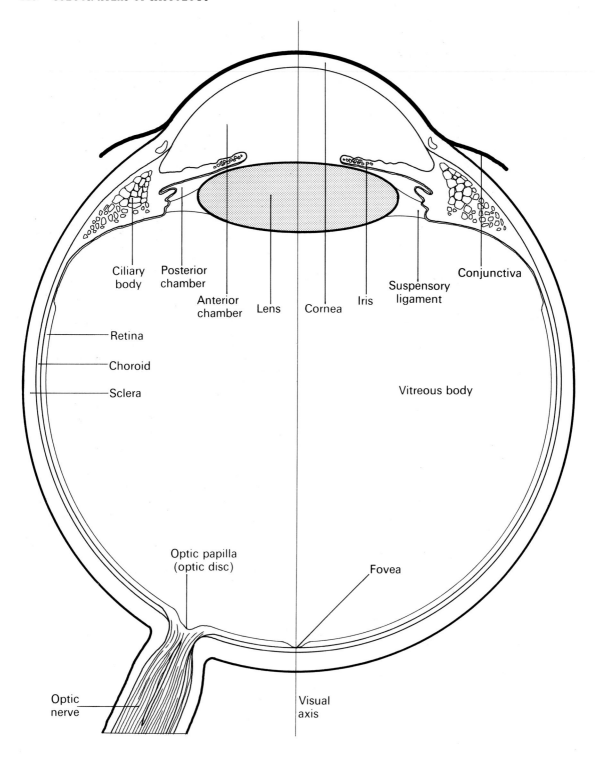

Ciliary body Posterior chamber Anterior chamber Lens Cornea Iris Suspensory ligament Conjunctiva

Retina

Choroid

Sclera

Vitreous body

Optic papilla (optic disc)

Fovea

Optic nerve

Visual axis

Fig. 13.19 The eye *(illustration opposite)*

The eye is a highly specialised organ of photoreception, a process which involves the conversion of light energy into nerve action potentials. The photoreceptors are modified dendrites of two types of cells, *rod cells* and *cone cells*. The rods are integrated into a system which is receptive to light of differing intensity; this is perceived in a form analogous to a black and white photographic image. The cones are of three functional types receptive to one of the basic colours, blue, green and red; they constitute a system by which coloured images may be perceived. The rod and cone receptors and a system of primary integrating neurones are located in the inner layer of the eye, the *retina*. All the remaining structures of the eye serve to support the retina or to focus images of the visual world upon the retina.

The eye is made up of three basic layers: the outer *corneo-scleral layer*, the intermediate *uveal layer* and the inner *retinal layer*.

(i) Corneo-scleral layer: The corneo-scleral layer forms a tough, fibro-elastic capsule which supports the eye. The posterior five-sixths, the *sclera*, is opaque and provides insertion for the eye muscles. The anterior one-sixth, the *cornea*, is transparent and has a smaller radius of curvature than the sclera. The cornea is the principal refracting medium of the eye and roughly focuses an image on to the retina; the focusing power of the cornea depends mainly on the radius of curvature of its external surface.

(ii) Uveal layer: The middle layer, the uvea or uveal tract, is a highly vascular layer which is made up of three components: the *choroid, ciliary body* and the *iris*. The choroid lies between the sclera and retina in the posterior five-sixths of the eye. It provides nutritive support for the retina and is heavily pigmented, thus absorbing light which has passed through the retina. Anteriorly the choroid merges with the ciliary body which is a circumferential thickening of the uvea. The ciliary body surrounds the coronal equator of the *lens* and is attached to it by the *suspensory ligament*. The lens is a biconvex transparent structure, the shape of which can be varied to provide fine focus of the corneal image upon the retina. The ciliary body contains smooth muscle, the tone of which controls the shape of the lens via the suspensory ligament. The lens, suspensory ligament and ciliary body partition the eye into a large posterior compartment and a smaller anterior compartment. The iris, the third component of the uvea, forms a diaphragm extending in front of the lens from the ciliary body so as to incompletely divide the anterior compartment into two chambers; these are known, somewhat confusingly, by the terms, *anterior* and *posterior chamber*. The highly pigmented iris acts as an adjustable diaphragm which regulates the amount of light reaching the retina. The aperture of the iris is called the *pupil*. The anterior and posterior chambers contain a watery fluid, the *aqueous humor*, which is secreted into the posterior chamber by the ciliary body. The aqueous humor is a source of nutrients for the non-vascular lens and cornea, and acts as an optical medium which is non-refractive with respect to the cornea. The pressure of aqueous humor maintains the shape of the cornea.

The large, posterior compartment of the eye contains a gelatinous mass known as the *vitreous body* consisting of so-called *vitreous humor*. The vitreous body supports the lens and retina from within as well as providing an optical medium which is non-refractive with respect to the lens.

(iii) Retinal layer: The photosensitive retina forms the inner lining of most of the posterior compartment of the eye. The retinal layer continues as a non-photosensitive epithelial layer which lines the ciliary body and the posterior surface of the iris.

The visual axis of the eye passes through a depression in the retina called the *fovea*. The foveal retina is the area of greatest visual acuity and contains only cone photoreceptors.

Nerve fibres from the retina converge to form the *optic nerve*. The retina overlying the *optic papilla (optic disc)* is devoid of photoreceptors and is thus referred to as the *blind spot*.

Within the bony orbital cavity, the eye is supported by a loose packing of fatty connective tissue. The exposed surface of the eye is protected by the eyelids. The mucus-secreting epithelium lining the inner surface of the eyelids is known as the *conjunctiva*. The conjunctiva and cornea are moistened and cleansed by watery secretions from the *lacrimal gland*, a small flattened gland located at the upper aspect of the eye. Modified sebaceous glands and apocrine sweat glands of the eyelid provide a superficial oily layer which inhibits evaporation. Tears drain to the inner aspect of the eye and thence into the nasal cavity via the *nasolacrimal duct*.

Fig. 13.20 Eye
(H & E ×5)

C – cornea
L – lens
I – iris
CB – ciliary body
O – optic nerve

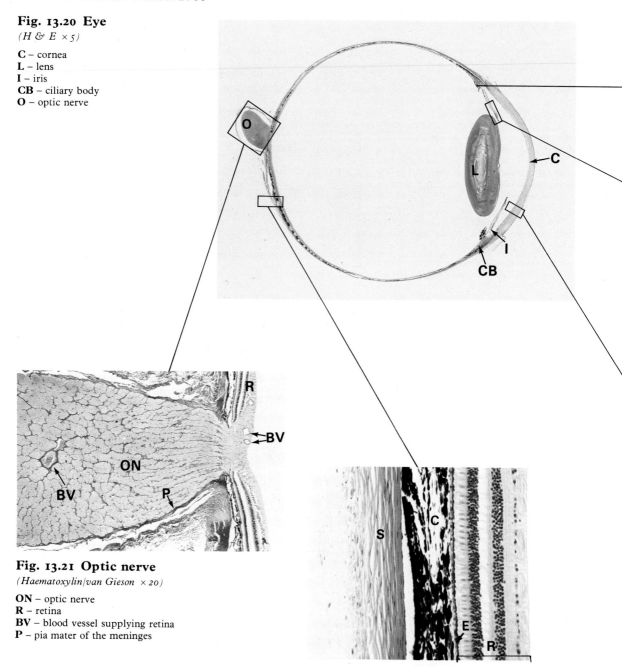

Fig. 13.21 Optic nerve
(Haematoxylin/van Gieson ×20)

ON – optic nerve
R – retina
BV – blood vessel supplying retina
P – pia mater of the meninges

Fig. 13.22 Wall of the eye
(H & E ×198)

R – retina
C – choroid; pigmented layer
S – sclera; dense regular connective tissue
E – pigmented layer of epithelial cells which form basal layer of the retina

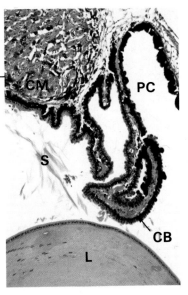

Fig. 13.23 Ciliary body and lens
(H & E × 128)

L – lens
S – suspensory ligament
CB – ciliary body; secretes aequeous humor
CM – ciliary muscle; adjusts lens for focusing
PC – posterior chamber

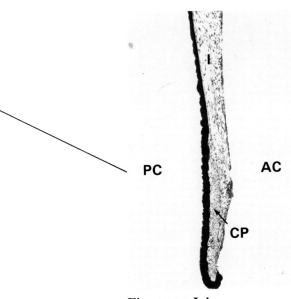

Fig. 13.24 Iris
(H & E × 20)

PC – posterior chamber of anterior compartment
I – iris; note pigment at posterior aspect
CP – constrictor muscle of pupil; dilator muscle cannot be distinguished
AC – anterior chamber of anterior compartment

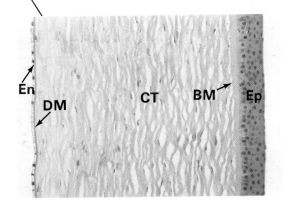

Fig. 13.25 Cornea
(H & E × 80)

Ep – outer stratified squamous epithelium
BM – Bowman's membrane; represents very thick basement membrane of outer epithelium of cornea
CT – dense regular connective tissue with no blood vessels
En – inner simple squamous epithelium
DM – Descemet's membrane; represents basement membrane of inner epithelium of cornea

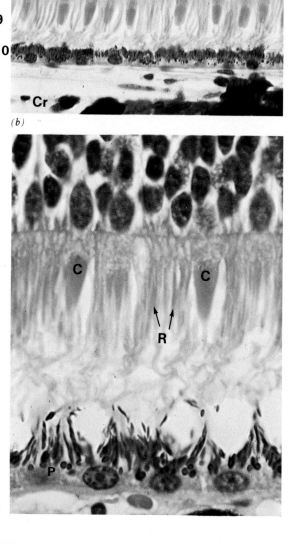

Schematic diagram labels (right side of diagram a):

Inner limiting membrane	①
Optic nerve fibres	②
Ganglion cell layer	③
Inner plexiform layer	④
Integrating bipolar cell layer	⑤
Outer plexiform layer	⑥
Cell bodies of rods and cones	⑦
Outer limiting membrane	⑧
Rods and cones	⑨
Pigment cells	⑩

(a)

Fig. 13.26 Retina

(a) Schematic diagram
(b) H & E × 640
(c) H & E × 1200

VB – vitreous body (contents of posterior compartment)
Cr – choroid; highly pigmented
R – rod receptor
C – cone receptor
P – pigmented epithelium

(b)

(c)

14. Skin

Introduction

The skin forms the continuous external surface of the body and in different regions of the body varies in thickness, colour and the presence of hairs, glands and nails. Despite these variations, which reflect different functional demands, all types of skin have the same basic structure. The external surface of skin consists of a keratinised squamous epithelium called the *epidermis*. The epidermis is supported and nourished by a thick underlying layer of dense, fibro-elastic connective tissue called the *dermis* which is highly vascular and contains many sensory receptors. The dermis is attached to underlying tissues by a layer of loose connective tissue called the *hypodermis* or *subcutaneous layer* which contains variable amounts of adipose tissue. Hair follicles, sweat glands, sebaceous glands and nails are epithelial structures termed *epidermal appendages* since they originate during embryological development from downgrowths of epidermal epithelium into the dermis and hypodermis.

The skin is the largest organ of the body, constituting almost one sixth of the total body weight; it has four major functions:

(i) Protection: the skin provides protection against ultraviolet light and mechanical, chemical and thermal insults; its relatively impermeable surface prevents excessive dehydration and acts as a physical barrier to invasion by micro-organisms.

(ii) Sensation: the skin is the largest sensory organ in the body and contains a variety of receptors for touch, pressure, pain and temperature.

(iii) Thermoregulation: in man, skin is a major organ of thermoregulation. The body is insulated against heat loss by the presence of hairs and subcutaneous adipose tissue. Heat loss is facilitated by evaporation of sweat from the skin surface and increased blood flow through the rich vascular network of the dermis.

(iv) Metabolic functions: subcutaneous adipose tissue constitutes a major store of energy, mainly in the form of triglycerides. Vitamin D is synthesised in the epidermis and supplements that derived from dietary sources.

Fig. 14.1 The skin

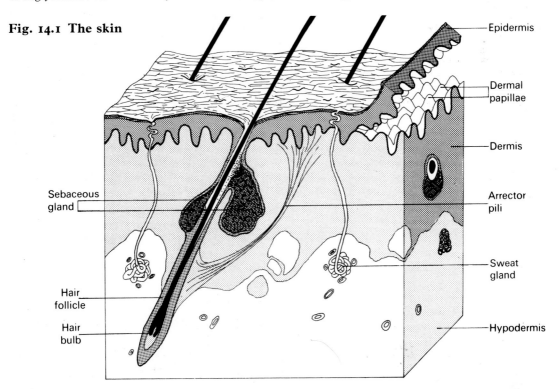

Fig. 14.2 The skin

Skin from fingertip: Masson's trichrome × 8

E – epidermis
D – dermis
H – hypodermis; containing adipose tissue and blood vessels
S – sweat gland
Pc – Pacinian corpuscle
Dt – sweat gland duct

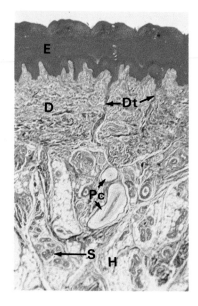

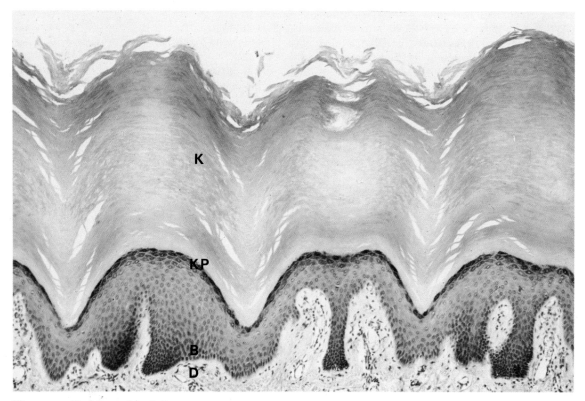

Fig. 14.3 Epidermis of fingertip

(H & E × 104)

K – keratinised layer
KP – keratin-producing layer
B – basal layer
D – dermis

Thyroid gland

The thyroid gland is a lobulated endocrine gland lying in the neck in front of the upper part of the trachea.

The thyroid gland produces hormones of two types:

(i) Iodine-containing hormones *tri-iodothyronine* (T_3) and *thyroxine* (T_4); T_4 is converted to T_3 in the general circulation. Thyroid hormone regulates the basal metabolic rate and has an important influence on growth and maturation particularly of nervous tissue. The secretion of these hormones is regulated by TSH secreted by the anterior pituitary.

(ii) The polypeptide hormone *calcitonin*; this hormone regulates blood calcium levels in conjunction with parathyroid hormone. Calcitonin lowers blood calcium levels by inhibiting the rate of decalcification of bone by osteoclastic resorption and by stimulating osteoblastic activity. Control of calcitonin secretion is dependent only on blood calcium levels and is independent of pituitary and parathyroid hormone levels.

The thyroid gland is unique among the human endocrine glands in that it stores large amounts of iodine containing hormones in an inactive form within extracellular compartments called follicles; in contrast, other endocrine glands store only small quantities of hormones in intracellular sites.

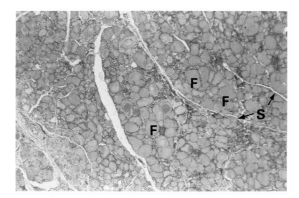

Fig. 15.8 Thyroid gland
(H & E ×8)

F – thyroid follicles; highly variable in size
S – delicate connective tissue septa which divide gland into lobules

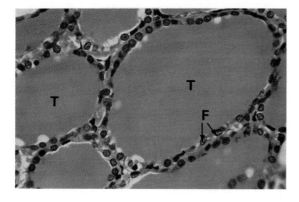

Fig. 15.9 Thyroid gland
(H & E ×128)

F – follicular cells; synthesise iodine containing hormones T_3 and T_4; note calcitonin is secreted by parafollicular cells which are scattered amongst follicular cells and in surrounding supporting tissues; parafollicular cells cannot be readily identified
T – thyroglobulin; storage form of thyroid hormone

Parathyroid gland

The parathyroid glands are small, oval endocrine glands closely associated with the thyroid gland. In mammals, there are usually two pairs of glands, one pair situated on the posterior surface of the thyroid gland on each side.

The parathyroid glands regulate serum calcium and phosphate levels via *parathyroid hormone (parathormone)*. Parathyroid hormone raises serum calcium levels in three ways:

(i) Direct action on bone by increasing the rate of osteoclastic resorption and promoting breakdown of the bone matrix.

(ii) Direct action on the kidney by increasing the renal tubular reabsorption of calcium ions and inhibiting the reabsorption of phosphate ions from the glomerular filtrate.

(iii) Promotion of the absorption of calcium from the small intestine; this effect involves vitamin D.

Secretion of parathyroid hormone is stimulated by a decrease in blood calcium levels. In conjunction with calcitonin, secreted by the parafollicular cells of the thyroid gland, blood calcium levels are maintained within narrow limits. Parathyroid hormone is the most important regulator of blood calcium levels and is essential to life, whereas calcitonin may only provide a complementary mechanism for fine adjustment.

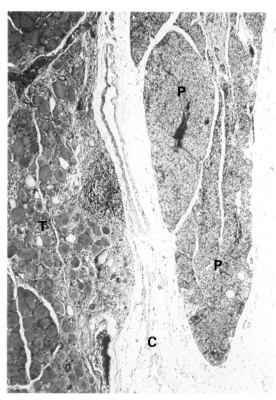

Fig. 15.10 Parathyroid gland

(H & E × 30)

P – parathyroid gland
T – thyroid gland
C – connective tissue capsule of thyroid

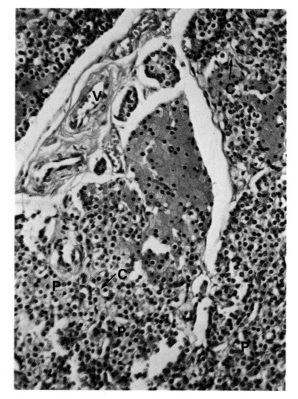

Fig. 15.11 Parathyroid gland

(H & E × 198)

P – chief or principal cells; thought to be active in parathyroid hormone synthesis and secretion
O – oxyphil cells; function not understood
S – supporting connective tissue septum
V – blood vessel
C – capillaries

Adrenal gland

The adrenal or supra-renal glands are small, flattened endocrine glands which are closely applied to the upper pole of each kidney. In mammals, the adrenal gland contains two functionally different types of endocrine tissue which have distinctly different embryological origins; in some lower animals, these two components exist as separate endocrine glands. The two components of the adrenal gland are the *adrenal cortex* and *adrenal medulla*.

(i) The adrenal cortex: the adrenal cortex has a similar embryological origin to the gonads and like the gonads, secretes a variety of *steroid hormones* all structurally related to their common precursor, *cholesterol*. The adrenal steroids may be divided into three functional classes; *mineralocorticoids* e.g. aldosterone, *glucocorticoids* e.g. cortisol and small amounts of *sex hormones*. The mineralocorticoids are concerned with electrolyte and fluid homeostasis. The glucocorticoids have a wide range of effects on carbohydrate, protein and lipid metabolism. Small quantities of sex hormones secreted by the adrenal cortex supplement gonadal sex hormone secretion.

(ii) The adrenal medulla: embryologically, the adrenal medulla has a similar origin to that of the sympathetic nervous system and may be considered as a highly specialised adjunct to the sympathetic nervous system. The adrenal medulla secretes the hormones, *adrenaline (epinephrine)* and *noradrenaline (norepinephrine)*.

The control of hormone secretion differs markedly between the cortex and medulla. Adrenocortical activity is mainly regulated by the pituitary trophic hormone ACTH, and release of each of the adrenal corticosteroid hormones is controlled by various other circulating hormones and metabolites. In contrast, the secretion of adrenal medullary hormones is directly controlled by the sympathetic nervous system. The function of the adrenal medulla is to reinforce the action of the sympathetic nervous system under conditions of stress; the direct nervous control of adrenal medullary secretion permits a rapid response to stressful stimuli.

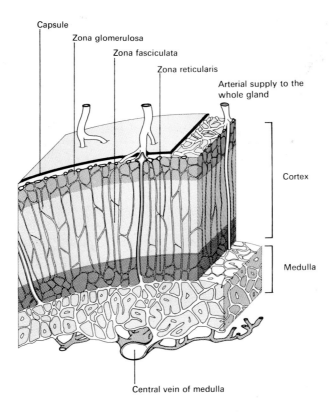

Fig. 15.12 Adrenal gland structure

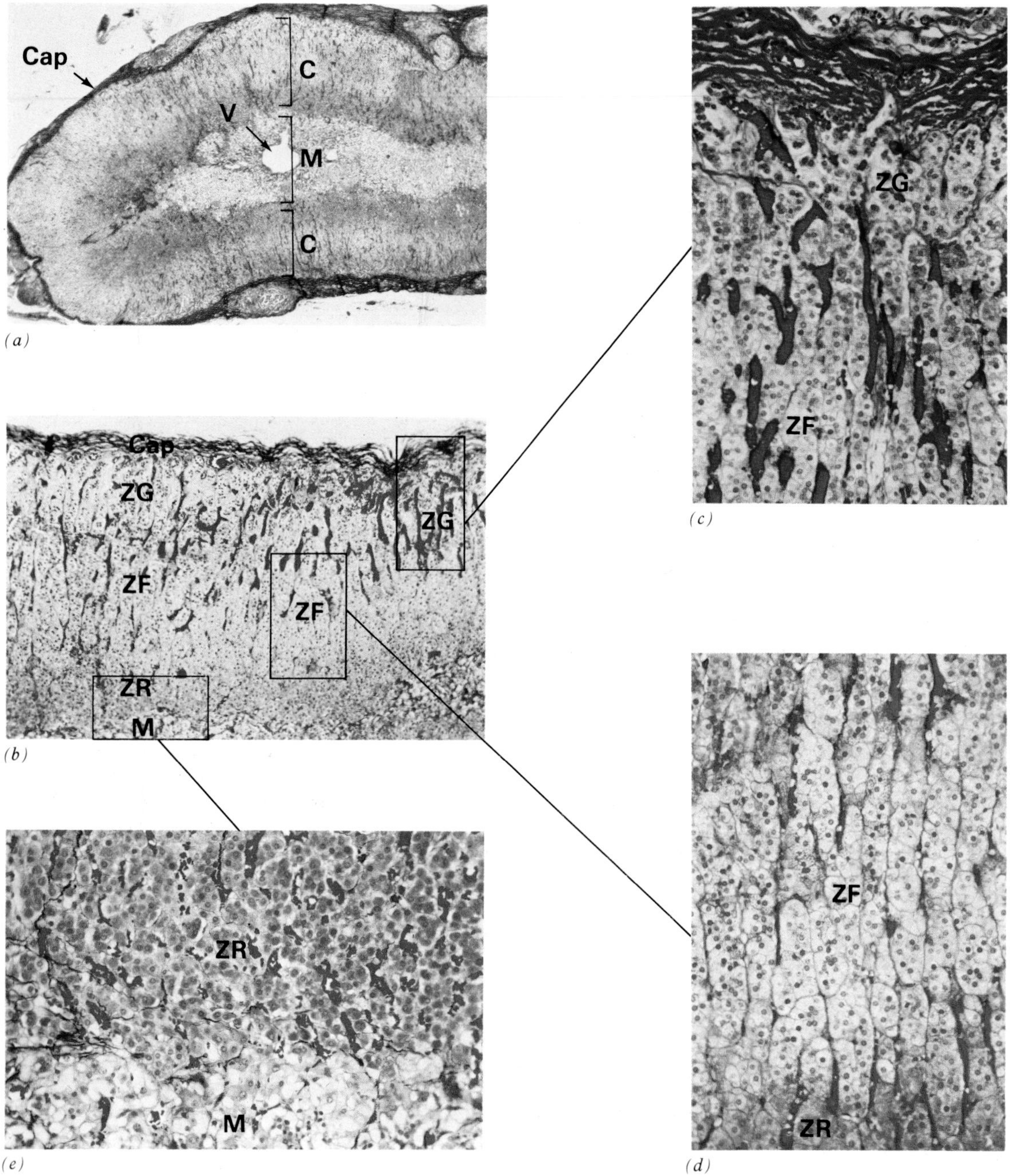

(a)

(b)

(c)

(e)

(d)

Fig. 15.13 Adrenal gland

(Azan (a) ×8 (b) ×20 (c) ×128 (d) ×128 (e) ×128)

C – cortex; divided into three zones
M – medulla; secretes adrenaline and noradrenaline
V – central vein of medulla
Cap – capsule of gland (collagen stains blue)

ZG – zona glomerulosa; secretes aldosterone
ZF – zona fasciculata; secretes cortisol
ZR – zona reticularis; may secrete small amounts of sex hormones

16. Female reproductive system

Introduction

The female reproductive system has the following major functions:

    (i) the production of female gametes, the *ova*, by a process called *oogenesis*;

    (ii) the reception of male gametes, the spermatozoa;

    (iii) the provision of a suitable environment for the fertilisation of ova by spermatozoa;

    (iv) the provision of an environment for the development of the fetus;

    (v) a means for the expulsion of the developed fetus to the external environment;

    (vi) nutrition of the newborn.

These functions are all integrated by hormonal and nervous mechanisms.

The female reproductive system may be divided into three structural units on the basis of function: the ovaries, the genital tract and the breasts.

The *ovaries*, paired organs lying in the pelvic cavity, are the sites of oogenesis. In sexually mature mammals, ova are released by the process of *ovulation* in a cyclical manner either seasonally or at regular intervals throughout the year. The cyclical ovulations are suspended during pregnancy. The process of ovulation is controlled by the cyclical release of gonadotrophic hormones from the anterior pituitary. The ovaries themselves have an endocrine function; they secrete the hormones *oestrogen* and *progesterone* which co-ordinate the activities of the genital tract and breasts with the ovulatory cycle.

The *genital tract* extends from near the ovaries to open at the external surface and provides an environment for reception of male gametes, fertilisation of ova, development of the fetus, and expulsion of the fetus at birth. The genital tract begins with a pair of *uterine tubes*, also called *oviducts* or *Fallopian tubes*, which conduct ova from the ovaries to the *uterus* where fetal development occurs.

Fertilisation of ova by spermatozoa occurs within the uterine tubes. The uterus is a muscular organ, the mucosal lining of which undergoes cyclical proliferation under the influence of ovarian hormones. This provides a suitable environment for implantation of the fertilised ovum. At birth, or *parturition*, strong contractions of the muscular uterine wall expel the fetus through the *cervix* into the birth canal or *vagina*. The vagina is an expansile muscular tube specialised for the passage of the fetus to the external environment and the reception of the penis during coitus. At the external opening of the vagina are thick folds of skin which constitute the *vulva*.

The breasts are highly modified sweat glands which, in the female, develop at puberty and regress at menopause. During pregnancy the breasts undergo structural changes in preparation for milk production or *lactation*.

In the non-pregnant state, the female reproductive system undergoes continuous cyclical changes from puberty to menopause. When ovulation is not followed by the implantation of a fertilised ovum, the proliferated mucosal lining regresses and a new ovulation cycle commences. In humans, the proliferated uterine mucosa is shed in a period of bleeding known as *menstruation*; the first day of bleeding marks the beginning of a new cycle of proliferation of the uterine mucosa which is known as the *menstrual cycle*. In humans, the menstrual cycle is usually of twenty-eight days duration and ovulation usually occurs at the midpoint of the cycle. The ovulatory and menstrual cycles are integrated by hormones secreted by the ovaries; ovarian hormones also promote cyclical changes in all other parts of the female reproductive system.

In other animals, the proliferated uterine mucosa is absorbed rather than shed and the female is receptive to the male only during the period of ovulation known as *oestrus* (or heat). The remaining part of the cycle is called the *dioestrus* and the whole cycle is known as the *oestrus cycle*.

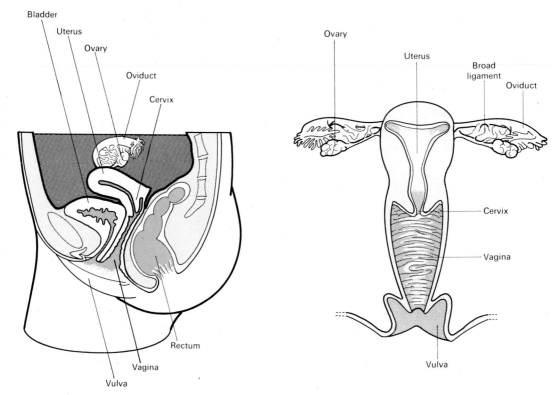

Fig. 16.1 Female reproductive system
(Sagittal section)

Fig. 16.2 Female reproductive system
(Coronal view)

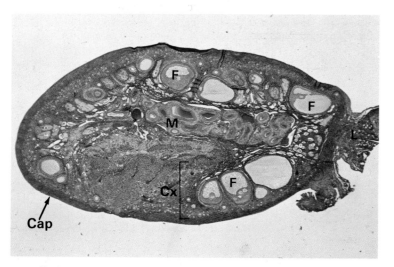

Fig. 16.3 Ovary

(Monkey: azan × 12)

Cap – ovarian capsule
Cx – cortex; contains follicles
M – medulla of ovary; highly vascular connective tissue
F – follicles in various stages of development

DEVELOPMENTAL EVENTS   DEVELOPMENTAL STAGE

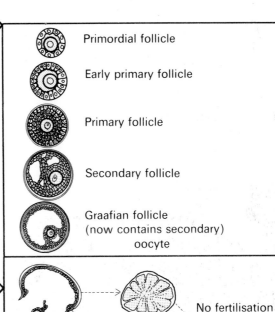

Primordial germ cells (oogonia)

Migration to ovarian cortex
6th week of fetal development

Multiplication by mitosis

Some oogonia develop the potential
to become mature female gametes.
Encapsulation by follicular cells
First stage of meiotic division
arrested

Primordial follicles containing primary oocytes

BIRTH

No further follicular development until
sexual maturity

SEXUAL MATURITY

Secretion of pituitary gonadotrophins
FSH & LH
Some primordial follicles develop
towards maturity with each ovarian
cycle

Increasing secretion of oestrogen
progressively inhibits release
of FSH and promotes LH release

Primordial follicle

Early primary follicle

Primary follicle

Secondary follicle

First meiotic division completed
Second meiotic division commences

High levels of oestrogen inhibit
FSH release and promotes large
release of LH

Graafian follicle
(now contains secondary)
oocyte

OVULATION

Progesterone secretion by
corpus luteum maintained by LH

No fertilisation

Corpus
luteum

No fertilisation
Degeneration

Corpus albicans

Inhibition of LH secretion by progesterone

FERTILISATION

After 3rd month
of pregnancy

IMPLANTATION

Corpus luteum of pregnancy maintained
by HCG secreted by developing embryo

Morula

Embryo

Corpus luteum
of pregnancy

Fig. 16.4 Development of human ova

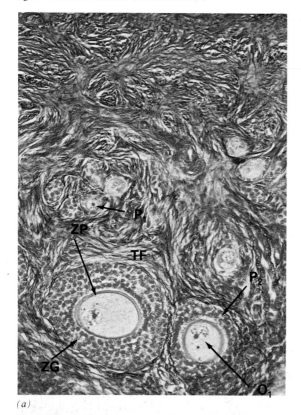

(a)

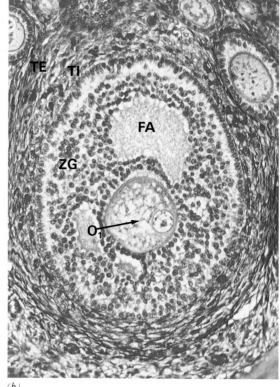

(b)

Fig. 16.5 Ovarian follicles

(Azan: (a) immature follicles × 120 (b) secondary follicle × 120 (c) Graafian follicle × 75)

P_1 – primordial follicle; contains primary oocyte
P_2 – primary follicle; primary oocyte now greatly enlarged
O_1 – primary oocyte; in process of first meiotic division
ZP – zona pellucida
ZG – zona granulosa
TF – theca folliculi; later differentiates into theca interna and theca externa
TI – theca interna
TE – theca externa
FA – follicular antrum; space containing follicular fluid
O_2 – secondary oocyte; second meiotic division now commenced
CR – corona radiata; still surrounds ovum after ovulation

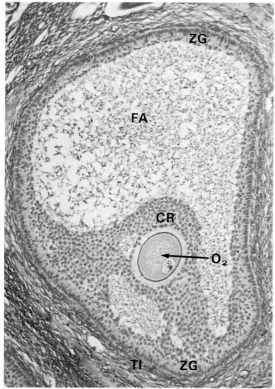

(c)

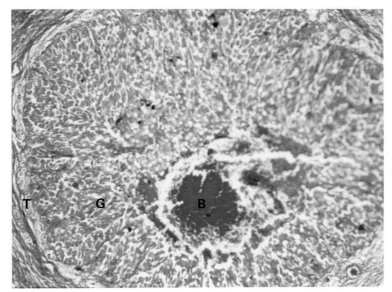

Fig. 16.6 Corpus luteum
(H & E × 75)

G – granulosa layer; formed from granulosa of Graafian follicle
T – thecal layer; derived from theca interna of Graafian follicle
B – blood clot remaining after ovulation

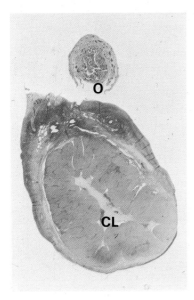

Fig. 16.7 Corpus luteum of pregnancy
(H & E × 3)

CL – corpus luteum; note depth of granulosa layer
O – oviduct

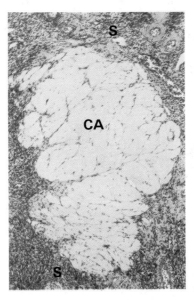

Fig. 16.8 Corpus albicans
(H & E × 20)

CA – corpus albicans; represents regressed corpus luteum
S – ovarian stroma

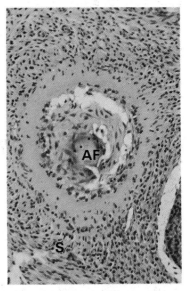

Fig. 16.9 Atretic follicle
(H & E × 128)

AF – atretic follicle; represents ovarian follicle which has failed to reach full development and has undergone degeneration
S – ovarian stroma

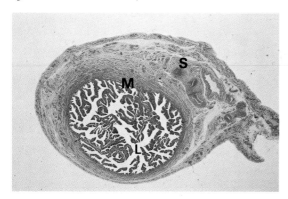

Fig. 16.10 Oviduct
(H & E ×10)

L – lumen; mucosa is folded into labyrinth
M – smooth muscle
S – surrounding highly vascular connective tissue

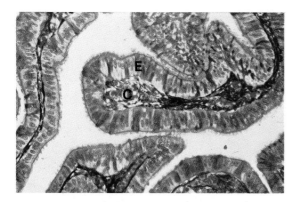

Fig. 16.11 Oviduct lining
(Azan ×128)

E – epithelium; composed of columnar ciliated cells and secretory cells (stained blue)
C – vascular supporting connective tissue

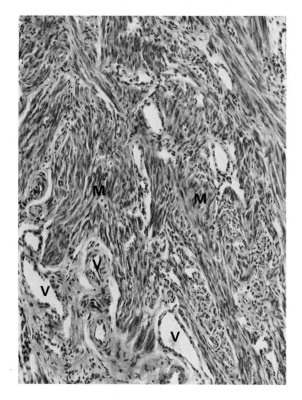

Fig. 16.12 Myometrium
(H & E ×198)

M – interlacing bundles of smooth muscle
V – blood vessels passing to endometrium

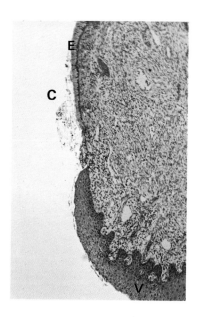

Fig. 16.13 Uterine cervix
(H & E × 128)

V – vaginal region of cervix; lined by stratified squamous epithelium
C – canal of cervix; lined by columnar ciliated epithelium **E**

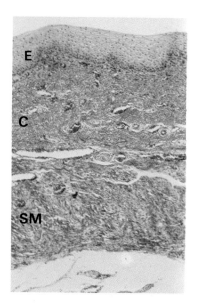

Fig. 16.14 Vaginal wall
(Masson's trichrome × 50)

E – epithelium
C – supporting connective tissue (collagen stained green), containing a large number of blood vessels
SM – smooth muscle

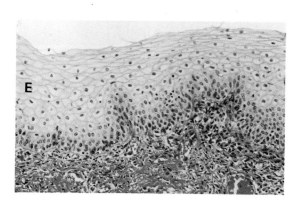

Fig. 16.15 Vaginal epithelium
(Masson's trichrome × 128)

E – stratified squamous epithelium; transudates glycogen-rich fluid; this is metabolised by vaginal commensal bacteria to produce lactic acid which lowers the pH of vagina to a level which inhibits growth of pathogenic micro-organisms.

The Hormonal Integration of the Ovarian
and Menstrual Cycles

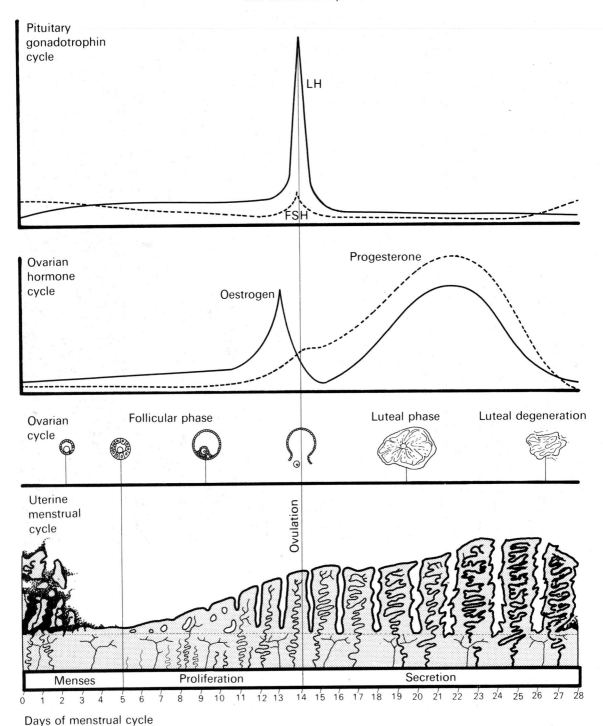

Days of menstrual cycle

Fig. 16.16 The hormonal integration of the ovarian and menstrual cycles

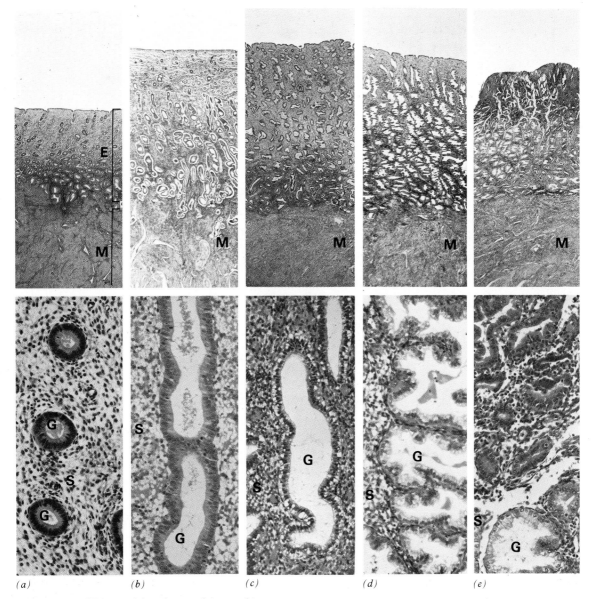

(a)   (b)   (c)   (d)   (e)

Fig. 16.17 Changes in the endometrium during the menstrual cycle

(H & E: Top row ×8, bottom row ×128; (a) early proliferative phase (b) late proliferative phase (c) onset of secretory phase (d) mid-secretory phase (e) onset of menstruation)

E – endometrium
M – myometrium
G – endometrial glands
S – highly vascular endometrial stroma

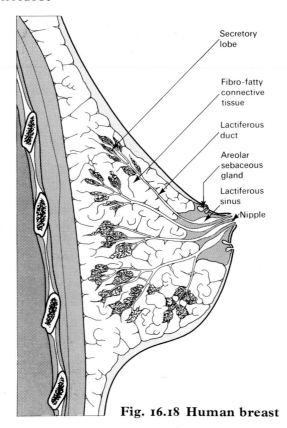

Secretory
lobe

Fibro-fatty
connective
tissue

Lactiferous
duct

Areolar
sebaceous
gland

Lactiferous
sinus

Nipple

Fig. 16.18 Human breast

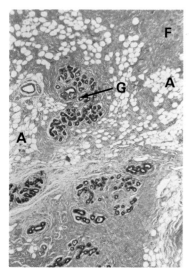

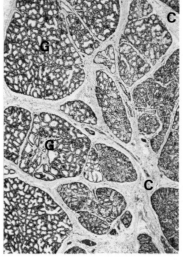

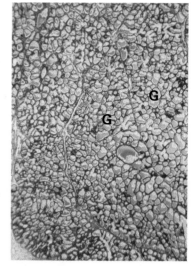

Fig. 16.19 Breast of woman of reproductive age

(H & E × 20)

G – glands; mainly ducts; acini develop during pregnancy
A – adipose tissue; comprises main bulk of breast
F – fibrous connective tissue

Fig. 16.20 Breast during pregnancy

(H & E × 20)

G – glands; duct system has proliferated and acini have formed at ends of ducts
C – connective tissue septa between breast lobules; note, adipose tissue is replaced by glands

Fig. 16.21 Breast during lactation

(H & E × 20)

G – glands; acini now filled with milk products and adipose tissue almost absent

17. Male reproductive system

Introduction

The male reproductive system may be divided into four major functional components:

(i) The *testes* or male gonads, paired organs lying in the scrotal sac, are responsible for production of the male gametes, *spermatozoa*, and secretion of male sex hormones.

(ii) A paired system of ducts, each consisting of *ductuli (vasa) efferentes, epididymis, ductus (vas) deferens* and *ejaculatory duct*, collect, store and conduct spermatozoa from each testis. The ejaculatory ducts converge on the *urethra* from which spermatozoa are expelled into the female reproductive tract during copulation.

(iii) Two exocrine glands, the paired *seminal vesicles* and the single *prostate gland*, secrete a nutritive and lubricating fluid medium called *seminal fluid* in which spermatozoa are conveyed to the female reproductive tract. Seminal fluid, spermatozoa and cells desquamated from the lining of the duct system comprise *semen*.

(iv) The *penis* is the organ of copulation. A pair of small accessory glands, *glands of Cowper*, secrete a fluid which prepares the urethra for the passage of semen during ejaculation.

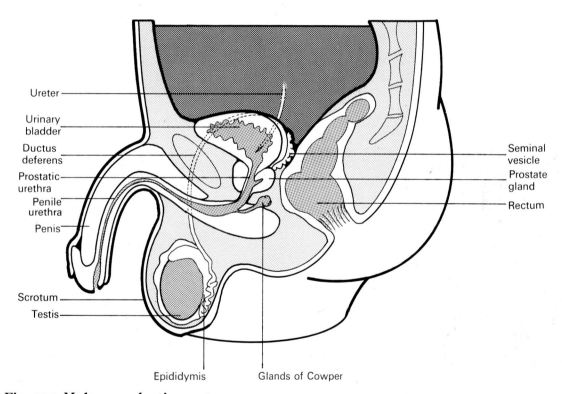

Fig. 17.1 Male reproductive system

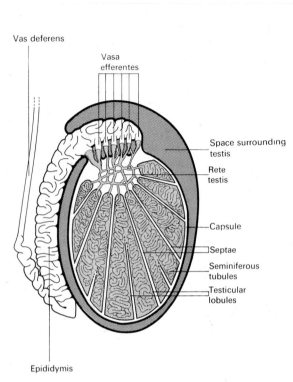

Fig. 17.2 Structure of testis

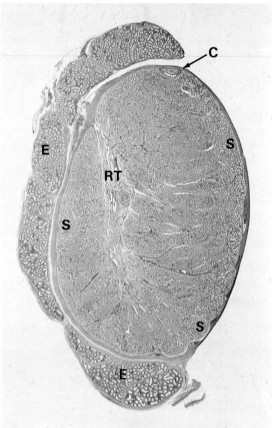

Fig. 17.3 Testis
(H & E × 3)

S – seminiferous tubules
RT – rete testis; collecting system for sperm from seminiferous tubules; sperm then pass via vasa efferentes to epididymis
E – epididymis; single highly convoluted tube; conveys sperm to vas deferens
C – capsule; dense connective tissue

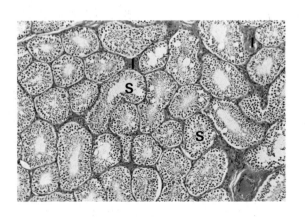

Fig. 17.4 Seminiferous tubules
(H & E × 50)

S – seminiferous tubules
I – intestitial spaces; contain Leydig (intestitial) cells and blood vessels

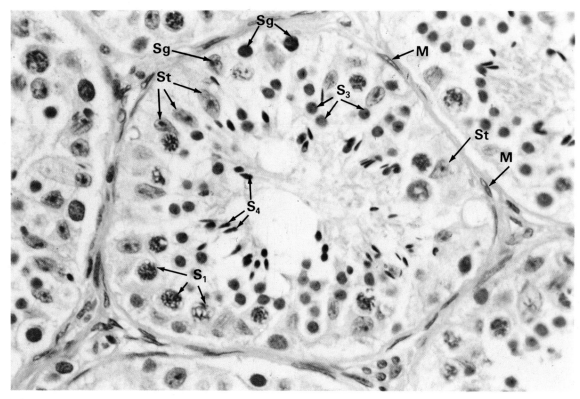

Fig. 17.5 Seminiferous tubule

(H & E ×640)

Sg – spermatagonia
S₁ – primary spermatocytes; undergoing first stage of
meiosis; no secondary spermatocytes are seen since this
second phase of meiosis occurs so rapidly
S₃ – spermatids; end products of meiosis; now undergo
development into spermatozoa

S₄ – spermatazoa
St – Sertoli cells; characteristic triangular nucleus and
prominent nucleolus
M – smooth muscle cells; these surround seminiferous
tubule and cause small local movements which propel
sperm, as yet non-motile, towards rete testis

Fig. 17.6 Interstitial cells of the testis

(Leydig cells: H & E × 480)

L – Leydig cells; secrete androgenic
hormones
C – interstitial capillary
S – seminiferous tubules

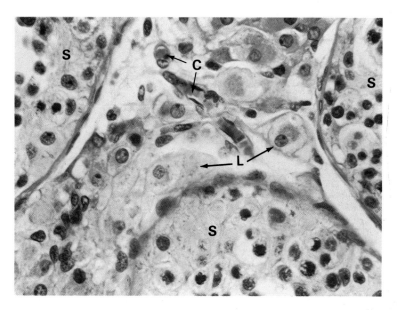

**Fig. 17.7 Male
reproductive system**

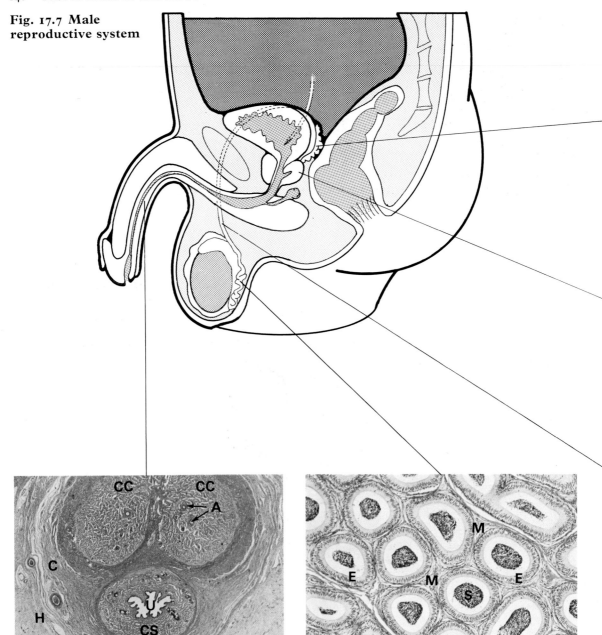

Fig. 17.8 Penis
(T.S: H & E ×8)

CC – corpora cavernosa
CS – corpus spongiosum; contains urethra
U – urethra
A – arterioles; supply blood to highly vascular erectile
tissue which make up corpora cavernosa and corpus
spongiosum
C – dense connective tissue sheath surrounding erectile
tissue
H – hypodermis; loose connective tissue underlying skin
of penis

Fig. 17.9 Epididymis
(H & E ×50)

S – spermatazoa; stored, undergo maturation, and develop
motility during passage through the extremely long
convoluted tubule which constitutes the epididymis
E – epithelial lining of epididymis
M – smooth muscle; contracts during ejaculation

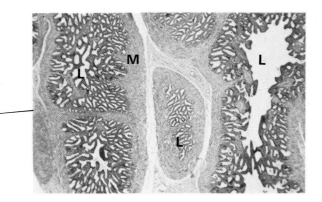

Fig. 17.10 Seminal vesicle
(H & E × 20)

L – labyrinthine lumen of seminal vesicle
M – smooth muscle; ejects secretions of gland during ejaculation

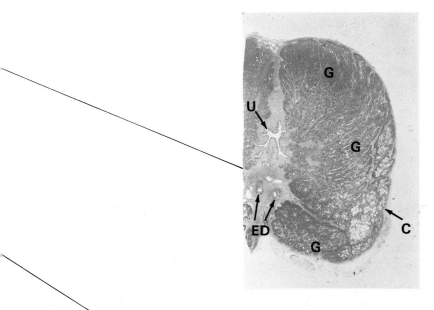

Fig. 17.11 Prostate gland
(H & E × 3)

G – prostate glandular tissue
U – urethra
ED – ejaculatory ducts
C – capsule of gland

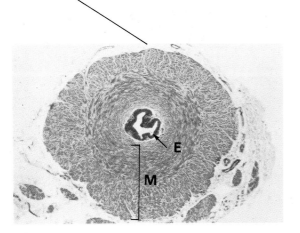

Fig. 17.12 Vas deferens
(H & E × 20)

M – thick smooth muscle made up of three layers; contracts during ejaculation
E – epithelial lining

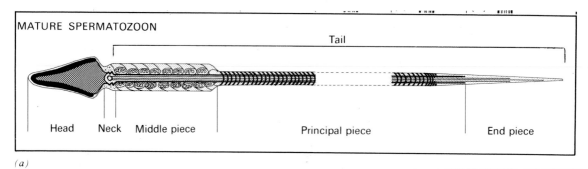

MATURE SPERMATOZOON

Tail

Head   Neck   Middle piece   Principal piece   End piece

(a)

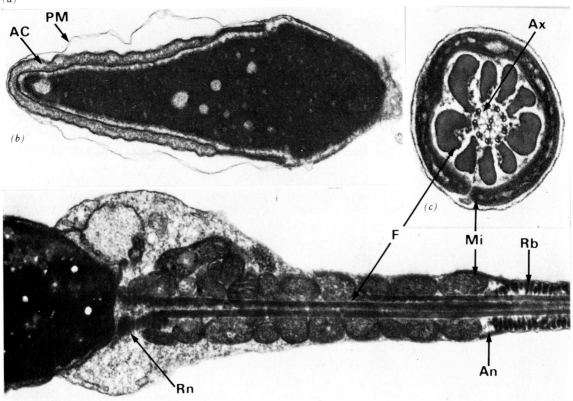

(b)

(c)

(d)

Fig. 17.13 Spermatazoa

(a) Schematic diagram (b) Head of sperm; L.S: EM × 14 000 (c) Neck, middle piece and principal piece: EM × 17 000 (d) Middle piece, T.S: EM × 48 000 (e) Semen: H & E × 800

PM – plasma membrane
AC – acrosomal cap
Rn – fibrous ring
C – cytoplasm
F – outer fibrils
Ax – axoneme
Mi – mitochondria
An – annulus
Rb – fibrous ribs
H – spermatazoon head
M – spermatazoon middle piece
T – spermatazoon tail
D – debris from reproductive tract

(e)

18. Immune system

Introduction

All living tissues are subject to the constant threat of invasion by disease-producing organisms, or *pathogens*, such as bacteria, viruses, fungi and multicellular parasites. Mammals have three main lines of defence against invading pathogens: protective surface phenomena, non-specific cellular responses and specific immune responses.

(i) Protective surface phenomena: in man, these provide a first line of defence. The skin constitutes a relatively impenetrable surface to most micro-organisms, unless breached by injury such as abrasion or burning. The sero-mucous surfaces of the body, such as the conjunctiva and oral cavity, are protected by a variety of anti-bacterial substances including the enzyme lysozyme, secreted in tears and saliva. The respiratory tract is protected by a layer of surface mucus which is continuously disposed of by ciliary action and replaced by goblet cell activity. The maintenance of an acidic environment in the stomach, vagina and to a lesser extent the skin, inhibits the growth of bacteria in these sites. When such defences fail to prevent access of pathogens to the tissues, the two other main types of defence mechanisms are activated.

(ii) Non-specific cellular responses: many types of pathogenic bacteria are spontaneously destroyed by the phagocytic cells of loose connective tissue after breaching an epithelial surface. Macrophages and neutrophils are the principal cells which carry out this function. Viral infections induce many cell types in the body to secrete an anti-viral substance called *interferon*, which disrupts viral multiplication within cells. Many pathogens evoke a multifactorial tissue response called *acute inflammation*; this process involves local changes in blood flow and attraction of blood-borne phagocytes to the site of pathogenic insult. When both protective surface phenomena and non-specific responses fail to check the invasion of pathogenic organisms, specific responses are activated, collectively known as the *immune response*.

(iii) Specific immune responses: many pathogens activate immune responses at the time of initial invasion, these specific responses are not, however, effective until a later stage. The non-specific responses are active in the interim period. The primary function of the *immune system* is the production of specific responses directed against specific pathogens. Thus, activation of the immune system involves recognition of characteristics peculiar to a particular pathogen; such characteristics are termed *antigens* since they generate responses directed at their own destruction which at the same time also destroy the pathogenic organism as a whole.

Lymphocytes are the functional units of the immune system and express their specific activity in two main ways. Firstly, some types of lymphocyte produce *antibodies* in response to the recognition of a particular antigen. Antibodies bind to antigens to promote destruction of antigen by a variety of mechanisms to be discussed below; the defence mechanism mediated by antibody is called the *humoral immune response*. Secondly, some lymphocytes are stimulated by antigens to produce a response in which circulating antibodies are not formed but in which lymphocytes and macrophages co-operate in the destruction of pathogenic organisms. This defence mechanism is called the *cellular immune response*. Although the humoral and cellular immune responses may occur separately, a single type of antigen often evokes both responses concurrently.

The cells of the immune system, principally lymphocytes, are disseminated throughout the body either as isolated cells, diffuse aggregations, or within the *lymphoid organs*. The principal *lymphoid organs* are the *thymus*, *lymph nodes* and the *spleen*.

Many of the mechanisms constituting the immune response are still widely disputed; however, most of the histological features of lymphoid tissue can be interpreted in terms of known immunological defence phenomena.

Fig. 18.1 The immune system

(illustration opposite)

This diagram summarises the principal mechanisms of the immune system. Lymphocytes are a heterogeneous population of cells all with a similar histological appearance. In functional terms, lymphocytes can be divided into a number of subpopulations, each with a different role in immunological defence.

Lymphocytes, like all other blood cells, are derived from a common stem cell in bone marrow. At some unknown point during lymphocyte development within bone marrow, each lymphocyte acquires the potential to recognise one specific antigen. These 'basic lymphocytes' are then released from bone marrow into the circulation and undergo further development in the lymphoid tissues to become mature, *immunocompetent* cells. Although basic lymphocytes have the potential to recognise specific antigens they must undergo either of two main maturation processes which determines the manner in which they will express their activity, that is via the cellular or humoral mechanism.

(i) The cellular immune response: basic lymphocytes destined to be involved in this type of response enter the thymus and undergo a series of changes before being released into the circulation; lymphocytes which mature in the thymus are called *thymus dependent* or *T lymphocytes*. From the circulation, T lymphocytes localise in the lymphoid tissues throughout the body, from which they then recirculate continuously via the blood and lymph circulations. The continuous recirculation of T lymphocytes has been interpreted as a 'quest for antigens'.

When a specific antigen is encountered in the tissues, the T lymphocytes which are programmed to recognise that particular antigen return to local lymphoid tissues and transform into *lymphoblasts*. Lymphoblasts then divide by mitosis to produce activated T lymphocytes which enter the circulation and migrate to the site of antigenic stimulation. Here they exert their destructive action in two main ways:

(a) Activated T lymphocytes produce a variety of substances, collectively called *lymphokines*, which attract and activate local and blood-borne macrophages. *Activated macrophages* possess greatly increased phagocytic activity which is directed towards destruction of antigen.

(b) Other activated T lymphocytes, called *killer T lymphocytes*, promote direct destruction of invading cells by a process termed *cytotoxic* destruction.

A small proportion of activated T lymphocytes remain in lymphoid tissues where they act as 'memory cells'; these are capable of mounting a more effective response on subsequent exposure to that particular antigen.

(ii) The humoral immune response: in mammals, those basic lymphocytes which will ultimately respond to antigens by producing antibodies, develop immunological competence in some as yet unknown organ. In birds, however, such lymphocytes mature in the *Bursa of Fabricius*, a lymphoid organ associated with the gastro-intestinal tract. Thus, these lymphocytes are called *Bursa-dependent* or *B lymphocytes*. Several 'bursal equivalents' have been suggested in mammals, including the tonsils, and lymphoid tissue of the intestines and appendix, but recent evidence suggests that the bone marrow itself may function as the mammalian bursal equivalent. By convention, the mammalian lymphocytes involved in the humoral response are called B lymphocytes.

Immunocompetent B lymphocytes, each programmed to recognise one particular antigen only, are released into the general circulation from which they seed the lymphoid tissues, mainly lymph nodes and spleen. In contrast to T lymphocytes, it is thought that most B lymphocytes do not continuously recirculate throughout the body but rather make contact with antigens taken up and processed by macrophages. When stimulated by antigen, B lymphocytes transform into *plasmablasts* which then divide to form antibody-producing cells called *plasma cells*. A proportion of plasma cells is thought to revert to B lymphocytes and remain in lymphoid tissue as 'memory cells'.

The secretion of antibody molecules by plasma cells takes place either within lymphoid tissue or at the site of antigenic stimulation. In the first case, antibodies are carried to the appropriate site by both the lymph and blood vascular systems.

The combination of antibody and antigen produces a complex which induces antigen destruction in three main ways:

(a) Simple neutralisation of soluble antigen: the complex is destroyed by phagocytosis.

(b) Opsonisation: some antigens are made more amenable to phagocytosis by combination with antibody. Antibodies which enhance phagocytosis are called *opsonins*.

(c) Complement activation: the combination of antibody and antigen may activate a system of plasma factors comprising the *complement system*. Activation of complement has three main effects. Firstly, some components of complement may act as opsonins; secondly, other components of complement attract neutrophils, thus acting as *chemotaxins*; thirdly, all nine components of complement act together to create holes in the plasma membranes of pathogenic cells resulting in cell death by osmotic lysis.

Antigens often initiate co-operative responses of both the cellular and humoral type. Furthermore, the co-operation of non-specific phagocytes is often necessary to produce the final destruction of antigen. Thus the response of lymphoid tissue to any particular antigen often shows histological features of cellular, humoral and non-specific responses.

This diagram summarises the main components of the immune response and the main tissue compartments in which they occur.

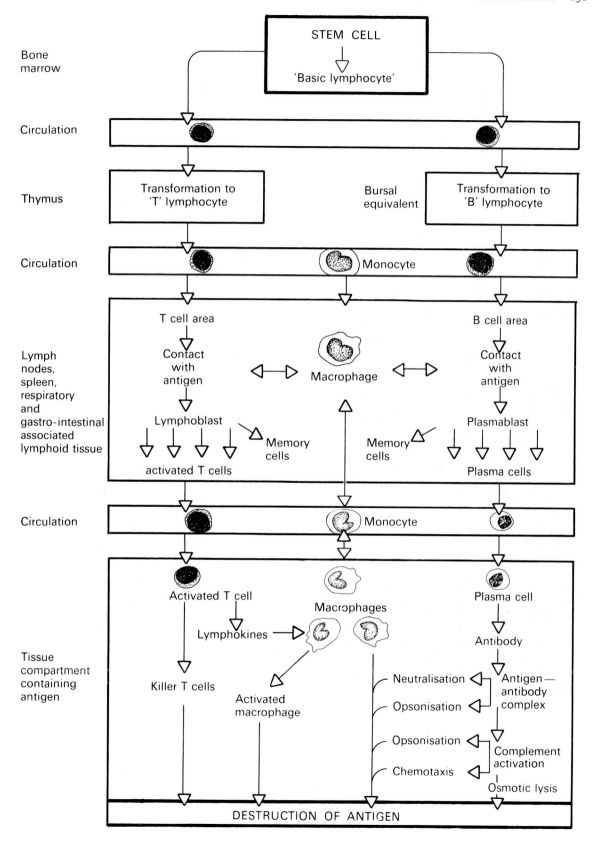

Thymus

The thymus is a lymphoid organ located in the anterior aspect of the thoracic cavity and lower part of the neck. During embryological development the thymus is the first lymphoid organ to appear; the major activity of the thymus takes place during childhood after which it gradually involutes such that, in human adults, the thymus is often impossible to differentiate from surrounding connective tissue. The thymus is derived from epithelial outgrowths of the primitive pharynx during embryological development; later, the primitive thymus becomes infiltrated by lymphocytes derived from blood forming tissue elsewhere in the developing embryo. The principal function of the thymus is the production of immunocompetent T lymphocytes by modification and proliferation of 'basic lymphocytes' produced by blood forming tissues. It has been postulated that the thymus also controls the development of lymph nodes and spleen during infancy by the production of a hormone called *thymosine*.

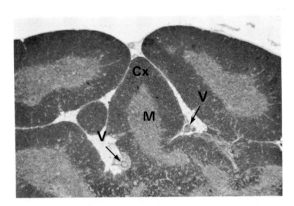

Fig. 18.2 Thymus
(H & E × 20)

Cx – thymic cortex
M – thymic medulla
V – blood vessels

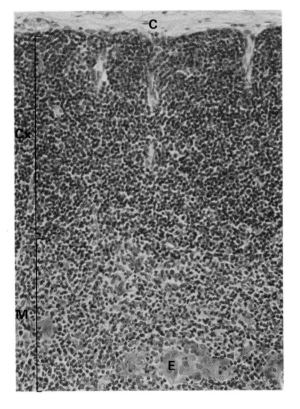

Fig. 18.3 Thymus
(H & E × 80)

Cx – thymic cortex; lymphocytes more closely packed than in medulla
M – thymic medulla
E – epithelial cells; these form a fine meshwork throughout the thymus which supports the lymphocytes
C – loose connective tissue capsule

Lymph nodes

Lymphocytes are distributed throughout the body where they are arranged in aggregations which exhibit various degrees of structural organisation. Isolated lymphocytes are found in most loose connective tissues and amongst epithelial cells, particularly the epithelium of the gastro-intestinal and respiratory tracts; in addition, large diffuse aggregations of lymphocytes are found in the walls of these tracts. The vast majority of lymphocytes are, however, located in encapsulated, highly organised structures called lymph nodes, which are interposed along the larger regional vessels of the lymph vascular system.

Three principal, interrelated functions occur within lymph nodes:

(i) non-specific 'filtration' of lymph by the phagocytic activity of macrophages;
(ii) storage and proliferation of B lymphocytes;
(iii) storage and proliferation of T lymphocytes.

T and B lymphocytes occupy different areas within lymph nodes; each area undergoes characteristic histological changes when appropriately stimulated by the presence of antigens. Even in the absence of overt disease, individuals are exposed to a wide range of antigenic stimulation from both within and without. Thus the histological appearance of a lymph node at any particular time will reflect not only the response to local antigenic stimulation but also the immunological status of the individual as a whole.

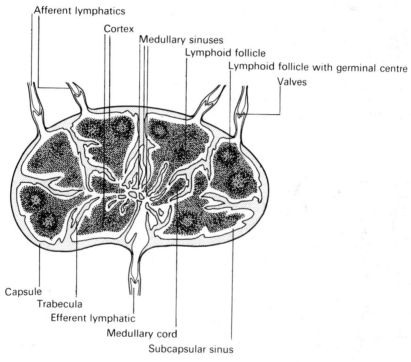

Fig. 18.4 Lymph node structure

Fig. 18.5 Lymph node
(H & E × 12)

C – capsule
Cx – cortex
T – trabeculae; supporting connective tissue
V – blood vessels
F – follicles
MC – medullary cords

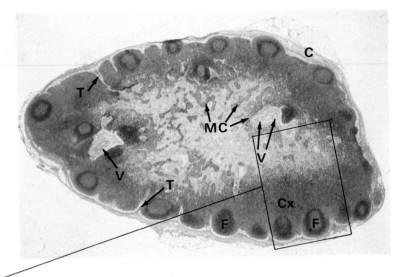

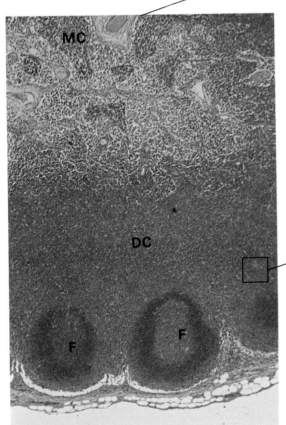

Fig. 18.6 B and T lymphocyte areas of cortex
(H & E × 30)

F – follicles with germinal centres; site of B lymphocyte proliferation
DC – deep cortex; site of T lymphocyte proliferation
MC – medullary cords; mature B lymphocytes and plasma cells predominate

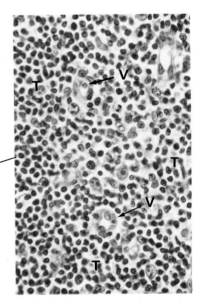

Fig. 18.7 T lymphocyte proliferation zone
(H & E × 320)

T – proliferating T lymphocytes
V – small blood vessels through which T lymphocytes pass into lymph node then back into the general circulation

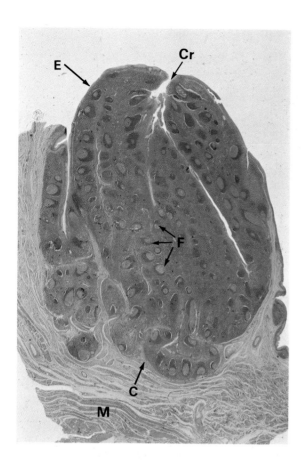

Fig. 18.8 Tonsil

(H & E ×6)

E – stratified squamous epithelial lining
C – connective tissue capsule
M – pharyngeal muscle
Cr – crypts which deeply invaginate the surface
F – lymphoid follicles; note pale stained germinal centres

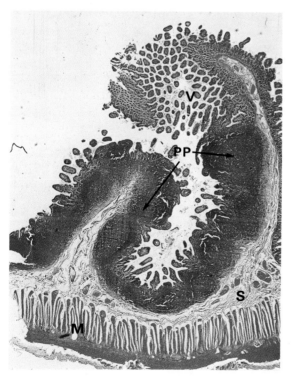

Fig. 18.9 Lymphoid aggregations in the small intestine (Peyer's patches)

(H & E ×16)

PP – Peyer's patches; note that there is no encapsulation but some germinal centre formation
M – smooth muscle layers
S – submucosal connective tissue containing blood vessels
V – villi cut in transverse, oblique and longitudinal sections

Spleen

The spleen is a large lymphoid organ situated in the left, upper part of the abdomen.

In man, the spleen has three main functions:

   (i) removal of particulate matter from circulating blood;

   (ii) production of immunological responses against blood-borne antigens;

   (iii) removal of aged or defective blood cells from the circulation.

In dogs and horses, the spleen also acts as a large reservoir of blood which can be mobilised if necessary. Despite its large size and important functions, removal of the spleen appears to have few deleterious effects on the body as a whole; its functions are assumed to be taken over by the liver and bone marrow.

The manner in which the spleen performs its functions, and many ultrastructural details, are still widely disputed; in many respects, however, the spleen may be considered analogous to a lymph node in which the lymphatic circulation is replaced by a blood circulation. The structure of the spleen provides for intimate contact to be made between blood and immunologically active cells just as the structure of lymph nodes facilitates the interaction of afferent lymph and lymphoid cells. Although it is well established that the spleen is involved in removal of aged or defective blood cells from the circulation, it is still not clear whether this is a purely mechanical process or whether immunological recognition plays an important role.

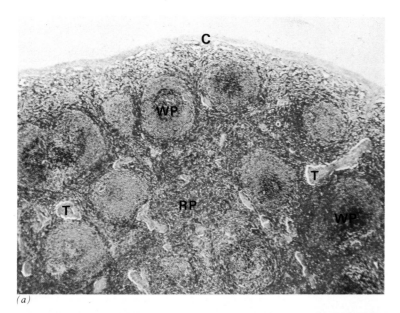

(a)

Fig. 18.10 Spleen

(H & E (a) spleen × 30 (b) white pulp with germinal centre × 80 (c) red pulp × 128)

C – tough connective tissue capsule
WP – white pulp; note some areas have prominent germinal centres as in (b)
RP – red pulp
A – arteriole of white pulp
T – trabeculae; convey larger blood vessels from capsule throughout the gland
B – cords of Bilroth
VS – vascular sinuses

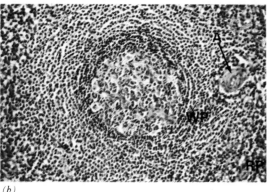

(b)

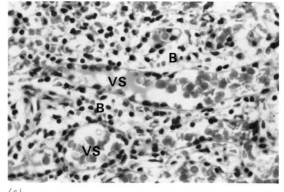

(c)

Index